women in organizations
barriers and breakthroughs

edited by

joseph j. pilotta

The Ohio State University

lawrence baum

kay deaux

sue dewine

mary anne fitzpatrick

tricia s. jones

linda l. putnam

Waveland Press, Inc.
Prospect Heights, Illinois

For information about this publication, write or call:

Waveland Press, Inc.
P.O. Box 400
Prospect Heights, Illinois 60070
(312) 634-0081

Dedication

For Judy

Contents

Acknowledgments

The essays presented in this volume are based on the workshop, "Communication and the Woman Manager: Barriers and Breakthroughs," held at Ohio State University on May 21-28, 1981.

The workshop was a special project of the Department of Communication's M.A. program in Communication Analysis and the Ph.D. track in Communication in the Public Interest. Sponsorship was provided by the Department of Communication, the College of Social and Behavioral Sciences and the Office of Continuing Education.

I wish to thank James Golden, Chairman, and William Brown, Graduate Director of the Department of Communication; Earl S. Brown, Dean of the College of Social and Behavioral Sciences; Joseph Oshins, Director, and Jeffrey Herold, Assistant Director of the Office of Continuing Education. Their commitment to public education and public issues made the workshop a success. A special thanks to the ninety workshop participants for encouraging the development of this book, and Patti Lind-Toledo and Ann Conrad for their assistance on the workshop.

Trust in Power in the Organization: An Overview[1]

Joseph J. Pilotta

Introduction

The effects of the women's movement, affirmative action programs, equal employment opportunities, and a general change in societal expectations of women and men have led to women being recognized as having a central place in organizational development. Organizations and women have started out on new ventures, without a clearly defined idea of what to expect.

It is not surprising that many women in the organization have found obstacles to successful communication between themselves and their staff or between themselves and their supervisors. Women have perceived some communication difficulties as unique to them. While there is truth to this claim, communication difficulties are a part of organizational settings.

In this book experts in the field of organizational communication explore the nature of some of the communication problems women face and examine them to see if they are unique to women. The strategies for overcoming difficulties are presented from the interdisciplinary perspectives of the authors.

---

[1]This essay is based on Niklas Lhumann's translated work entitled *Trust and Power*, (New York: John Wiley, 1980).

Kay Deaux discusses the "fear of success" theme which is the hypothesized motive of what prevents women from achieving in the manner in which men do. However, research suggests that the "fear of success" is neither a pervasive motive nor is it the exclusive possession of women. Men and women approach situations anticipating consequences that result from their actions, and both will choose *self-presentation* strategies that maximize the probability of attaining positive results. Therefore, women's achievement behavior can be seen to result not only from characteristics of the woman, but from the general context and specific policies of the organization.

Tricia Jones discusses the topic of sexual harassment in terms of situated behavior which may be considered harassing in the organizational setting. Sexual harassment has been shown to result in emotional, mental, and physical stress for the person who has been the *object* of harassment. This stress in turn is reflected in an organizational loss of productivity and worker satisfaction. The consequences of sexual harassment are presented with practical recommendations for effective and appropriate responses to a harassment incident. The recommendations include a general program of action available to individuals as an aid to avoid personal and organizational consequences of sexual harassment.

Lawrence Baum's essay points out that, traditionally, individuals in business and college organizations have had few legal rights regarding their treatment by people with *authority* over them. The government, now, has established a body of rights for employees and students and has given relationships within the organization a legal quality. A significant example of the "legalization" process is the adoption of laws that prohibit discrimination on the basis of sex. An examination of the actual impact of laws concerning sex discrimination indicates that these laws have made a difference, but their impact is limited by important organizational constraints.

Linda Putnam focuses on the development and evolution of cyclical relationships between supervisor-subordinates as well as on peer-related dilemmas which entrap women in self-perpetuating and destructive role conflicts. These dilemmas are troublesome to organizational women who already feel trapped in the paradox of *competition* through *cooperation*. The cooperative-competitive dilemma in organizations requires alternative message strategies for managing and resolving organization *conflicts* and for breaking the vicious cycle.

There has been a plethora of research in the past 10 years examining male-female differences in communication style and outcome. Mary Anne Fitzpatrick places this research in a comprehensive framework by examining the issues of *communicative competence*. Success in any organizational structure is hypothesized to depend, at least to some degree, on the individual's ability to communicate effectively to accomplish his/her interactional goals. Fitzpatrick offers a model for the accomplishment of interaction goals by both male and female communicators.

Sue Dewine offers an essay on breaking through the communication barriers in organizations by providing a practical model for building professional alliances. The process of building professional alliances is called *networking*. Networking "links" people to each other as career resources and supports and helps others find resources they need. Networking reduces isolation and increases *participation* and *self-confidence*.

The orientation of these essays reveals two fundamental dimensions of societal and organizational communicative action. These dimensions are the practices of Trust and Power. The concern with trust and power as communicative practices are central concepts to any form of organizational development in modern society. *Women in Organizations* is concerned with the development of self-knowledge in the face of power. The motivation for self-knowledge, which we will call *trust*, demands that women in organizations cannot ignore power. To ignore power assures one's own powerlessness. Alternatively, if women understand the basis of trust and the relations of power in an organization, women improve the quality of their self-knowledge and can become *empowered* themselves.

The remainder of this introductory essay will discuss a *general* theoretical and practical overview of the nature of trust and power. This essay is written in broad strokes to encourage thinking about the organization in a new way without being mired down in the jargon of a more detailed analysis. The essays which follow deal with various aspects and approaches to the trust and power themes. Central to these essays are the following concepts: self-presentation, competition-cooperation, conflict-resolution, communicative competence, participation and self-confidence (which are concerned with organizational trust), the harassed as "object," authority, legalized relationships and conflict (which pertain to the power concept).

What Is Organizational Trust?

Trust is necessary for compliance with organization rules. Without trust individuals would not be able to live in and with the various aspects of organizational complexities. Trust is a communication relationship which secures and stabilizes future action or expectations which means that "things" will generally occur the way you think they will. Trust in the organization conditions the manner in which men and women can anticipate the future. To be able to trust in the organization means that the individual is familiar with the organizational climate and with other men and women in the organization. It is familiarity in the organization which allows individuals to *anticipate* or trust that they can anticipate how others will view and act toward them. Trust signals that contingencies exist in the organization which means there are certain harms or benefits which occur with any expected action.

The foundations of trust in the organization, which has a personal side, are adjusted according to the prospects and conditions for the presentation of self. The problem of forming trust relationships must be solved gradually. It is necessary to an organization to promote behavioral choices for individuals. Human action in an organization must be perceived as personally determined in order for trust to be created. One cannot stick strictly to their behavioral roles in the organization, for they will not be trusted. Rather, individuals must initiate trusting behavior and go beyond the boundaries of expected role behaviors.

Trust is necessitated by interdependence in the organization, which is the condition for cooperative and fair competition relationships, but trust is created and sustained because it is possible that the cooperative partner can abuse the trust. The possibility to abuse trust necessitates mutual commitment to working relationships. One cannot *demand* the trust of others, trust can only be offered and accepted. It is a learning process, which can only be completed when the person to be trusted has had opportunities to betray that trust and yet has *not* used those opportunities.

If individuals stay in their role and organizations demand strict role behavior, then the role relationships are risk-free and there are hardly any available starting points for the development of individual trust in the organization. Therefore trust is a fundamental communicative-ethical process.

Women are ready to trust if they possess an inner-security, a self-confidence. Their readiness to trust needs cognitive security. While trusting itself is an ethical problem, in order to be able to trust, women must be able to anticipate others' as well as organizational actions.

Is Trust Based on Stability?

Some people believe that stability in the organization cannot be built upon a changing environment. However, research has shown that insecure expectations are learned and are held on to more firmly than secure ones. Secure expectations collapse at a first disappointment while uncertainties are more stable because they contain the opposite expectation as well. The insecure expectation as well as the secure one become organizationally stereotyped which minimizes our expectations from being refuted. Expectations are highly immune from external refutation in that they incorporate with their own contradictions. Therfore, trust is a balancing of the secure and insecure expectations. This is what is meant by being an open person and able to take risks.

The readiness to trust comes from this inner assurance of self-presentation in all situations; for even trust is an act of self-presentation. Self-presentation relies on knowing the boundaries of a situation. The sources of the assurance of self-presentation are various. They range from rational abilities of imagination and quick reaction to status, education, experience or success.

But fundamental readiness to trust *always*, but always, rests on the organization which confers trust, by creating the conditions which can allow it to happen. In other words, an organ-

ization must be able to take into account how it structures
ethical relationships in the work place. Mutual commitment
and cooperation are necessary for productive and satisfying
working relations which are only accomplished through trust.

Power

Classically, power has not been based on a selective process
of communication, but rather, on a causal form of communication. That is, the causal form of communication tries to con-
ceive power as a cause that brings about specific effects, or
generally as the ability to make others act in a way they would
not have chosen of their own free will. This is a transitive,
hierarchical conception of power. It excludes the possibility of
reciprocal power relations.

The causal form of power-communication views the power-
holder's calculations as essentially producing a causal
sequence of events that are determined by fixed needs. It
prevails in cases of conflict. In addition, causal power is
viewed as a kind of possession that can be gained or lost and
that remains constant in the organization. In other words,
every loss of power means a gain of power for an opponent.

Power is a symbolically and generalizable capacity to condition, regulate, and motivate certain choices on the part of
others. The communication of power has as its goal to make the
premise of any decision the premise of your decision.

Communication only happens if one understands how a
certain message is chosen to be delivered. The primary communication medium is language. *The communication of power
operates when symbols employed in the communication
motivate or urge the acceptance of other person or persons
choices, making the acceptance the object of their
expectations.* The subordinate is motivated to implement the
decision because there are other possibilities. Subordinates'
acceptance of the decision takes place because they are aware
that there are well established alternatives which are unpleasant for the participants and which therefore need to be
avoided. For example, in the case of women, discrediting is
used. Power operates through this generalized form of communication which we call influence.

Influence is a way of reducing the number of tasks to be performed in an organization. Influence presumes a shared meaningful orientation. Influence is generalized in three directions:

(1) It is independent of individual characteristics.

(2) It is independent of where it is experienced.

(3) It is independent of who experiences it.

Accepting influence is the same as *making a choice*. Individuals accept influence because one has accepted influence on other matters. Also, individuals accept influence because others accept it too. The ability to generalize is called authority and the symbolic ability to influence is power.

Organizational and Personnel Power

Organizational power is relative to the membership or personnel as a whole.

(1) Organizations are formed if it is taken for granted that individuals can join or leave it and rules are developed for individuals to make this decision; therefore,

(2) Organization assumes that members' roles are contingent.

(3) Organizational power is more sensitive to short-term situations, therefore, they stabilize contingent rules and make them official.

Organizational power rests on the competence to give official directives, the recognition of official directives is a condition to membership which can sanction dismissal. The actual power in organizations depends, for the most part, on influencing the careers of individuals.

Organizational power limits are based on the shortage of usable personnel, while the limits of personnel power are in the shortage of attractive positions in the organization. The sanction of organizational power, dismissal, is used infrequently. It is a negative alternative. Sanctioning through personnel power occurs more frequently. Personnel power consists mainly of preferring other applicants for a position and may only appear as a negative sanction to those rejected. Therefore, personnel

power is *based* more on the anticipation and attribution of
intentions.

Organizational power increases with the formal framework
of rules. But personnel power tends to be decreased if it is tied
to formal rules for the occupation of positions, criteria for job-
analysis or standardized personnel evaluation. But, such rules
are used as power mechanisms or excuses for making one's
negative treatment appear as another's positive one.

Organizational power and personnel power together can
increase one's own power. Both forms of power are brought
together under the hierarchy of subordinates. For instance, if
the decision-making ability concerning personnel is taken away
from the immediate superior, who alone can operate effectively with personnel, then she/he can retain influence over decisions through personnel assessment, also a source of power.

Strain on a power-holder in an organization can be exploited
by others as their own source of power, if the power-holder's
position does not provide discretion for action or non-action.
One can have access to a power-holder's power by withholding
information, which in turn insulates the individual from the
power-holder. Also, if the power-holder does not have the discretion to act (or non-act), then one can count on the power-
holder seeking *consensus* because the power-holder will have
to rely on cooperation.

The power accrued by subordinates is obtained individually.
It results from situations and is dependent on personal initia-
tive. Subordinates *taking over power* is not based on a simple,
reversal, because subordinate power rests on their positions
as subordinates and on the impotence of power-holders who in
the organization lack discretionary power. Subordinates have
to beware of trying to access power by renouncing the power of
their superior and in turn attempting to take over the reins.
Often there is an attempt to systematize or legitimatize the
power   of   subordinates   in   the   organization.   This
legitimatization   is   sanctioned   by   the   organization   and
encouraged by the slogans of "participation" and "equality."
Committees of subordinates are formed to give input into the
decision-making process. But, this is a management of communication distortion or manipulation under the pretense of
participation. It is essentially reorganizing the power which the

employees already have. This deprives the subordinates of their power base which lies in them being subordinates.

Women must take a look at the rhetoric of "democratizing" the work place, and heed the directive of Mary Parker Follet, "The division of power is not the thing to be considered, but that method of organization which will generate power."[2]

A Model for Communication Empowerment in the Organization[3]

Communication in the organization requires information dissemination which engenders trust. Organizational communication must address its employees by satisfying four practical conditions.

(1) Information must be clear and comprehensible in the organization,

(2) Sincere,

(3) Appropriate to the situation, and

(4) Accurate.

These conditions of communication address four organizational vulnerabilities:

(a) Vulnerability of person's comprehension of issues, particularly clear attribution of responsibility for certain decisions.

(b) False assurance given through experts in organization.

(c) The vulnerability to management by consent, e.g., legitimacy claims by supervisor-top-down communication only.

(d) Vulnerability to misrepresentation of facts.

In other words, how women respond to anticipated threats of misinformation will depend, in part, upon what is understood

---

[2]Follett, Mary Parker, "Power" in Henry C. Metcalf and Lyndall Ururich (eds.) *Dynamic Administration: The Collected Papers of Mary Parker Follett*, (London: Southampton, 1941), p. 111.

[3]See Habermas Jurgen, *Communication and the Evolution of Society*, (Boston: Beacon Press, 1979).

as the effective sources of power which can influence and create misinformation. To ask, "What are the sources of effective misinformation which need to be anticipated and countered?" becomes a practical organizational question. What are the types of power faced by women in organizations? How does power work, and how is it limited or vulnerable?

Generally, informing and misinforming women in the organization is an exercise of power which is management through the communication of·

(a) comprehension (or obfuscation),

(b) assurance (or false assurance),

(c) consent (or manipulated agreement), and

(d) knowledge (or misrepresentation).

In order for the possibility of development to occur for individuals in the organization these four conditions for assessing genuine communication must be constantly checked and monitored to avoid manipulated communication. The discovery of manipulated communication engenders mistrust, yet the discovering of manipulated communication can be a source of *empowerment* for women.

Internal Barriers

Kay Deaux

Still in the world today, and in organizations in particular, some unfortunate truths persist. These "facts of life" can be stated quite simply:

(1) Many people don't think women can make it.

(2) Many people don't think women have made it when they have.

(3) And if women do make it, and if that performance can not be denied, spurious reasons are often found for their success.

For the woman in the organization, these external barriers are pervasive and often seem insurmountable. Research in academic laboratories has provided ample support for what many women know to be true — that they are not being judged on the same basis that men are. Consider the following results of laboratory studies. When people are asked to describe a typical man, a typical woman, or a successful manager, a clear pattern emerges. The successful manager is viewed as quite similar to the average man, and both are seen to be quite different from the average woman. Who is the personnel manager likely to hire for the executive training program?

When people are asked to estimate how well a man or woman will do on a variety of jobs, they expect that the man will do better — particularly if it is a job or field that has traditionally been identified with men. When people are asked to evaluate the performance of a man or a woman, they tend to

11

rate the performance of the man as better — particularly if it is
in a traditionally male field. Doesn't everyone want to hire the
person that they think will do the best job?

When asked to explain why a person has done a job well,
people also reach different conclusions, depending on whether
that person is a man or a woman. For men, success is most
often seen to result from the man's ability. For women, that
same performance will often be attributed to luck, to the simplicity of the job, or to a particular burst of effort on that one
occasion. Who would you want to promote to the next level?
Someone who had real ability, or someone who had been successful through no "fault" of their own?

These are the kinds of external barriers that women encounter. Although many of the above statements are based on
laboratory research, the corporate world offers hundreds of
examples of their reality base. The case of Mary Cunningham
provides one clear example.[1] Her name became a household
word in 1981, as she was promoted at the age of 29 to executive
vice-president for strategic planning of Bendix. Within days of
the announcement of her promotion, readers of daily news-
papers were treated to photographs of Mary Cunningham,
descriptions of her hair and her clothes, information about her
estranged husband, and, most significantly, speculation about
her relationship with her mentor, the Chief Executive Officer of
Bendix Corporation. Why this flurry of interest? Mary
Cunningham was not the youngest manager to assume a major
position in a U.S. corporation; nor was she the first to have a
mentor to accelerate her progress. But most of these other
young stars were men, and the explanations for their accel-
erated rise were different. They were "boy wonders" and she
was of suspicious character. They were "on the rise" and she
was "on the make." The evaluations of Mary Cunningham's
performance were different, and the explanations for her success were different. So, too, was the outcome: Mary
Cunningham resigned in the face of pressure from Bendix.

Although opportunities for women have increased substantially in recent years, there are still a great many barriers re-

---

[1] I give credit to Virginia O'Leary for the development of this example.

maining. Some laws have changed but others remain. Further-more, the laws themselves may provide handy explanations for those people who are reluctant to acknowledge female compe-tence. "We hired her because we were getting pressure from the government," many a company official has been heard to state, with the clear implication that better-qualified men were left standing at the door of the employment office. Although affirmative action policies and government legislation may well have been necessary to facilitate women's hiring, the very existence of these policies can create another tangential ex-planation that diminishes the perceptions of women's capabil-ities.

These barriers, important as they are, are external to the woman herself, while the title of this contribution suggested a concern with internal barriers. For reasons that I hope to demonstrate, these two domains are related. Many of the stereotypes and assumptions about women that society makes have been internalized by the woman herself. She too may believe what other people say and even more frequently think. And even if she surmounts these internal barriers, she must still take action in the face of the external barriers that persist.

Internal Barriers: Expectations and Performance

As we have seen, people generally expect women to do worse than men, they tend to evaluate the performance of women less favorably, and they are more inclined to find spur-ious reasons for the success that women do have. These same three patterns can be found in the behavior of women them-selves, constituting a powerful internal barrier to achieve-ment.

In the first case, women often expect to do more poorly than men. In a large number of laboratory experiments, men and women have been asked to state their expectations for per-formance on a variety of tasks and in a variety of situations. Most often, the men predict better performance than do the women. These lowered expectations are particularly characteristic of women when the setting is ambiguous and when feedback about previous performance is not provided. For this reason, it may be especially important for women to demand feedback in an organization. Frequent objective assessments may help the woman get a more accurate picture of her past performance, thus helping her to predict future performance more accurately.

One might question whether women, with their tendency to expect to do more poorly, are in fact any less accurate than men when actual performance is taken into account. The truth is that both sexes seem to be in error: women generally do better than they think they will, while men tend to fall short of their expressed expectations. Thus, neither sex has cornered the market on accuracy. However, for reasons that will become clear shortly, overestimation may be a more profitable option than underestimation.

Not only do women often expect to do worse than do men, but they also tend to undervalue the performance that they have done. Thus in studies conducted both with college students and with first-level supervisors in a retail sales corporation, women have rated their performance less favorably than men. In a similar vein, research by Brenda Major has shown that when women and men work on a job for the same amount of time, men will reward themselves significantly more pay for that job than will women, despite the equivalence of their efforts. The reverse holds true as well: when men and women are given a set amount of money and asked to work for as long as they think is appropriate, women work longer for the same amount of money than do men.

Each of these behaviors may reflect a tendency on the part of women to undervalue their own accomplishments. Expecting to do worse and evaluating their actual performance less favorably, they may come to believe that they are simply worth less on the marketplace than men, thus incorporating into their own belief system the stereotypes of others. Additional evidence for this lowered evaluation on the part of women can be seen in a common work situation: asking for a starting salary. In a series of studies, Brenda Major has found that among M.B.A. students, for example, women will state a lower desired salary figure than will men. More significantly, her research has shown that simulated employers will award salaries that correspond to these requests. In other words, the more you request, the more you get (within reasonable limits, of course).

These results are paralleled by actual employment data. Recent analyses reported in the *Wall Street Journal,* for example, show that the average female M.B.A. graduate in fact does receive a lower starting salary than the average M.B.A. male graduate. Such findings suggest that pay discrimination may at least in part be under the woman's control, and that breaking down internal barriers can improve the situation.

Still another internal barrier that may act to impede women's progress is the kind of explanations that they use to explain their own performance. In the case of external barriers, we saw that people will explain a man's success by reference to his inherent ability, while relying on more transitory or external factors such as task simplicity, chance, or effort to explain the woman's success. Women often do the same thing to themselves. Thus while the successful man is most apt to claim that his innate ability is responsible, the woman is more apt to look to other factors, such as help from or the favor of others, the non-challenging nature of the job, or the fact that she tried very hard. And again, explicit affirmative action policies of the organization may be seen by the woman as the cause of her being hired or being promoted to a higher-level job. Echoing the comments of others, she may feel that her gender rather than her ability contributed to the positive outcome.

Explanations for failure to perform well have also been shown to differ between women and men. Men, while claiming ability as a reason for their success, eschew inability as a possible cause for failure. Now they are the ones who look to external causes outside themselves for an explanation. Or if taking some of the blame upon themselves, men point to a lack of effort as the cause, thus allowing themselves to believe that by working harder, success will be inevitable. In contrast, women more often turn to inability as a cause for their failure, and in turn are more likely to believe that success can not be achieved because of this inherent lack of ability.

Of course not all men use only self-serving attributions, nor do all women use only self-deflating explanations. Nevertheless, the trends are pronounced, and to the extent they are characteristic of the individual woman, they may serve as a potent internal barrier. Such explanations may most critically serve as a barrier when they are not ends in themselves. Thus, to the extent that what one believes about a past experience influences choices for the future, then the explanations and beliefs become powerful indeed.

Research by Madeline Heilman and Richard Guzzo has shown that the employer who believes that an employee's performance was due to ability will reward that performance with both a raise and a promotion. If effort is believed to be the major factor in performance, then a raise is considered appropriate but a promotion is not. Finally, if other factors external to the employee are considered most important, then neither a raise nor a promotion is given. To the extent that individuals explain their performance in the same terms, we might anticipate some similar consequences. For example, what if you feel that your performance was due to help from a colleague? Would you be willing to go into your supervisor's office and ask for a raise? In contrast, what if you believed that you really had the ability necessary to grow with the company? Is a request for a promotion more likely? It seems probable that such explanations are indeed influential. To the extent that the individual believes "I was just lucky on that assingment," advancement may be slow to come.

Internal Barriers: Achievement Motivation and the Fear of Success

So far we have considered the behaviors that surround a specific performance or assignment: the expectations, the evaluation of the performance, and the explanations offered for success or failure. Yet there is another factor that people have claimed is a much more serious barrier to women's success, and that is the general motive for achievement. As used by psychologists, motives are internalized drives or urges, often learned early in life, that continue to initiate and direct behavior in later life. Among the most widely-studied of such hypothesized motives is the need for achievement, reflecting, among other factors, the premium this country puts on individual accomplishment and success. People who have strong achievement needs are presumed to strive continually for excellence, attempting to accomplish projects and achieve goals. Achievement motivation, as studied by David McClelland and others, is assumed to contribute to the entrepreneurial spirit, and programs have been developed to encourage the growth of this motive in future managers, both in this country and throughout the world.

The history of research on achievement motivation has been a male history. Nearly three decades ago, when this research began, a decision was made to focus attention on the achievement behavior of men. There were a couple of reasons for this decision. First of all, men's behavior followed the predictions of the theory while women's seemed inconsistent with theoretical predictions. Rather than change their theory, investigators decided to select their subjects more carefully. In other words, they eliminated women from the studies. Secondly, looking at the real world, people saw more evidence for what they believed to be achievement among men—the political leaders, the officers of corporations, the scientists and artists—and thus they concluded that achievement was primarily a male endowment.

Yet even in the early studies there was evidence that women possessed needs for achievement in the same degree as did men, and in recent years investigators began to pursue the question of why women were not achieving more. Perhaps the most popular explanation has been the concept of fear of success, developed by Matina Horner. (It should be noted that Matina Horner herself has evidenced no fear of success! Shortly after completing her doctoral work on this aspect of achievement, Horner assumed the presidency of Radcliffe College, a position she still holds today).

What is fear of success? According to Horner, fear of success is a motive that is learned early in life, as is the need for achievement. People who develop this particular type of motivation will, despite the achievement needs they may have, avoid success in a variety of situations. But why would anyone find success aversive? In many cases, Horner suggests, the consequences of success may be negative. Through early experience, an individual may learn that success can be followed by rejection, by jealousy on the part of others, and by other negative reactions. According to Horner, this motive is particularly strong in women, who learn to expect rejection by men, loss of femininity, and other similar effects if they succeed. In other words, because the society's stereotype suggests that women should not be competent—at least not in traditionally male fields—negative sanctions may be applied to the woman who does in fact succeed in a traditionally male environment.

The woman who fears success is not without achievement needs. Indeed, Horner suggests that it is primarily women who have strong achievement aspirations who will be able to see what negative consequences might result. Feeling the need to accomplish and having the ability to do so, they may still hold back for fear of rejection. Furthermore, Horner suggests that this motive comes into play most strongly in the presence of men and in the face of direct competition. Such an internal barrier would seem to provide a convincing explanation for the apparent lack of accomplishment of women, relative to men, in the arenas of politics, commerce, academics, and the arts.

Research has provided some support for the influence of fear of success. For example, women who score high in fear of success have been found to have less commitment to a career, and to use self-defeating strategies in achievement situations. In an interesting follow-up study to Horner's original work, Lois Hoffman found that women who had shown a high degree of fear of success in 1964 were, in 1974, more likely to be married and to be mothers, and less likely to have full-time careers. Furthermore, there was suggestive evidence that these same women, when pursuing careers that began to eclipse the success of their husbands, were quite likely to become pregnant, thus reducing, at least temporarily, their career development.

Yet although it is important to recognize the nature of this internal barrier to some women's success, it is also important to put this motive in its proper context. First of all, fear of success is not innate, being born into women at the time of their conceptions. Rather, it is the reality of the external world—the instructions, the experiences, and the reinforcements—that fosters the development of this motive. In truth, women are more likely than men to experience negative consequences for achievement, and their learning thus mirrors the reality of a world that still discriminates. In this regard, it is interesting to note that black women generally show less fear of success than do white women. Perhaps, because more black women have worked in the past and because more of these women have had to work from economic necessity, negative sanctions have been far less common in their experience.

A second issue is what kind of success is feared. In Horner's original studies, people were asked to describe a situation in which a student was at the top of a first-year medical school class. Women were asked to describe the consequences for a hypothetical "Anne," while men were to depict the situation of a hypothetical "John." Under these conditions, women described far more negative consequences than did men, leading Horner to conclude that women were more likely than men to suffer from a fear of success. Yet what if the situation is changed? What if both Anne and John are in nursing school, a field traditionally dominated by women? In this case, we find that far more men describe negative consequences than do women. This latter research suggests that fear of success may not be a global motive, applying equally to any situation in which success is possible. Rather, people—both women and men—may fear success when the situation is one that traditionally has not been viewed as appropriate for their sex. Thus the man in nursing, elementary education, or secretarial fields may have fears as strong as the woman in management, construction, or the steel industry, and both do so for some accurate reasons. In looking at a single field—management, for example—women may appear to have more fear of success than men, and thus fear of success is indeed an internal barrier that should be taken into account. That is not to say, however, that fear of success is either exclusive to women, general to all endeavors, or without a basis in reality.

Furthermore, if the environment proves the expectations wrong, fear of success may not rear its detrimental head. Thus the male partner who is supportive and proud of his spouse's success can make fears of rejection and loss of femininity seem groundless. Similarly, coworkers and supervisors who make it clear that performance rather than gender is the critical issue can also allay fears of success. Most people, after all, will avoid negative consequences. The woman who does so in achievement settings may be considered "afraid of success." However, if the negative consequences for her successful performance vanish, we will probably find that fear of success has evaporated as well.

The Interplay of Internal and External Barriers

Many people would like to place the responsibility for women's limited presence and decelerated progress within organizations on other persons, on the corporation, on the society at large. Others prefer to level the charge at the woman herself, pointing to faults, deficiencies, or inabilities on her part. In truth, both of these positions are oversimplified. The fact is that neither set of barriers exists in a vacuum. Internal barriers exist in large part because of the external barriers that have been set up for generations. And, conversely, external barriers increase their longevity by virtue of the internal barriers that prevent women from exercising their full potential. To understand how both sets of barriers can be reduced in size, and eventually eliminated, it is important to understand how they reinforce each other.

We have seen how a set of beliefs regarding the characteristics and potential of women managers exists. Furthermore, these beliefs are not only descriptive, but they are prescriptive as well, in other words, the message conveyed is not only that women generally *are* this way or the other, but that they *should* be that way. It is almost impossible for a woman not to encounter such beliefs as she attempts to enter the corporate world. More detrimental, however, is the fact that these beliefs do not exist in the abstract. Rather people act upon these beliefs in their dealings with women.

In laboratory research, Mark Snyder and his colleagues have shown that an individual who believes he is interacting with a woman will make different choices than if he believes he is interacting with a man, independent of whom the hidden partner actually is. In a similar fashion, the upper-level manager who believes that a woman is capable only of routine assignments may assign only that kind of job, preventing her from even attempting the more challenging assignments. At the same time, this upper-level manager may give his male trainee far more challenging assignments, operating under the belief that men are more capable of such tasks. Assuming that both the man and the woman do reasonably well in their given assignments, the rewards will still be different. Success in a challenging job is worth more to the organization than success in a routine job, and the woman may never have the opportunity to prove that she is capable.

Sometimes these beliefs are displaced onto others under the guise of pragmatics. For example, the marketing director may believe that his male and female account managers are equally capable, yet still feel that his major clients would not accept a woman in charge of their business. Thus this director may give men the most important accounts and relegate women to the less consequential ones, even though he personally has little doubt that the woman could be equally effective.

Whatever the underlying reasons for their choices, supervisors who take these actions are constructing formidable barriers to the success of women managers. For we are all influenced, to a greater or lesser extent, by the forces of the situation. Behavioral scientists have long been aware of the importance of "self-fulfilling prophecies." Defined most simply, this phrase refers to the fact that if we believe something to be true, it tends to happen. Set in an organizational context, if the supervisor believes that women are only capable of certain jobs, then she may in fact only do those certain jobs — and the prediction becomes reality. Further, employees who are treated as if they do not have the capability to make major decisions will in time not attempt to make major decisions.

Here is where the internal barriers come into play. I have done research in the steel industry, for example, where there have traditionally been very few women employed in the higher-paying, higher status craft occupations. One could easily argue that women were discriminated against, not allowed to enter these particular jobs. At the same time, however, it can be shown that until recently very few women applied for these jobs. It seems quite probable that many supervisors believed that women were not qualified for these positions, and hence recruitment strategies were directed at males only. Consequently, women themselves probably came to believe that the craft jobs were not appropriate for them, or that they could not learn the necessary skills. Yet when the situational forces shifted somewhat — in this case, because of consent decrees between the union, the industry, and the government — women were encouraged to apply for crafts and many did so. The woman who ten years ago would have considered a craft occupation out-of-bounds, now applied for training, completed it, and liked the occupation. The weakening of external barriers led to a weakening of internal barriers.

Thus the woman in the organization must take stock, both of her own beliefs and expectations, and of the beliefs and expectations of those whose opinions are critical to her development and success. Breaking down only one set of barriers will rarely prove satisfactory. The interplay between the two sets perpetuates the process, and the influence of both barriers must be analyzed, modified, and eventually eliminated. The ultimate breakthrough is of course elimination of the barriers. But the first breakthrough must be the recognition that they exist, and the determination to weaken their influence, both in oneself and in the world around.

Sexual Harassment in the Organization

Tricia S. Jones

Organizational members are commonly faced with situations which might be considered sexually harassing; for example, sexual jokes and innuendos, unnecessary touching, or even overt propositions for sexual intimacy. While the problem of sexual harassment is important for both male and female employees, women are more commonly the victims of such behavior. In light of the prevalence and consequences of sexual harassment employees in any organization should become informed about the nature of sexually harassing behaviors in order to combat harassment successfully in their place of employment.

Sexual harassment has become a major personnel issue in the last decade. Due to the recency of this recognition the identification and prevention of sexual harassment may be idiosyncratic. The courts and individual organizations are still attempting to define harassment and thereby identify the behaviors which constitute harassment. This continuing definitional confusion has made it difficult to establish effective avenues of redress for sexual harassment victims. To date appropriate individual and organizational responses to the problem of sexual harassment are still being determined through a process of trial and error.

In light of the seriousness of sexual harassment for both individuals and organizations this article presents a review of information concerning the prevalence and consequences of harassing behaviors, discusses some legal implications of this behavior, and recommends appropriate individual responses and organizational policies which may discourage harassment. Although this article focuses primarily on the female victim of harassment the information presented is equally important for male targets of sexual harassment. For their own protection organizational members of either sex should be informed about and prepared to deal with incidents of harassment in their place of employment.

Sexual Harassment: What Is It?

There is no widespread agreement on the individual behaviors that are inherently harassing. Most definitions of harassment attempt to define this behavior in terms of its context through specifications of the relationship between the perpetrator and target of harassment, indications of general categories of "harassing" behavior, and the effects of such behavior on the victims of these incidents. While there are numerous definitional disagreements most current definitions of sexual harassment agree that harassment involves behavior of a sexual nature that is unwelcome to the recipient.

A review of some contemporary definitions of harassment exemplify areas of definitonal disagreement. Some authors, such as Lin Farley in her book *Sexual Shakedown,* maintain that harassment is "unreciprocal male behavior which asserts a woman's sex role over her function as a worker."[1] A more general definition offered by the U.S. Office of Personnel Managements describes sexual harassment as deliberate or repeated unsolicited verbal comments, gestures, or physical contact of a sexual nature that is unwelcome.[2] The most encompassing and legally relevant definition posited to date is supplied by the recent Equal Employment Opportunity Guidelines on Sexual Harassment. The Guidelines define harassment as:

1. Unwelcome sexual advances

---

[1]Lin Farley, *Sexual Shakedown: The Sexual Harassment of Women on the Job* (New York: McGraw-Hill, 1979), p. 14.
[2]Robert L. Woodrum, "Sexual Harassment: New Concern About an Old Problem," *S.A.M. Advanced Management Journal,* 46 (1981), p. 23.

2. Requests for sexual favors (including requests between members of the same sex)
3. Other verbal or physical contact of a sexual nature if:
   a. The person's employment depends upon submission
   b. Acceptance or rejection of the conduct affects any employment decision concerning the harassed person, and,
   c. The conduct interferes with the person's work performance or creates an intimidating, hostile, or offensive work environment.[3]

Each of these definitions emphasizes a specific contextual variable. Farley's definition focuses on the nature of the harasser, portraying sexual harassment as sex discrimination of women. The OPM definition attempts to define harassment by presenting general categories of harassing behaviors without specification of the nature of the harasser or the effects of harassment. The apparently comprehensive defintion offered by the EEOC Guidelines identifies harassment largely in terms of the consequences of harassment for the target. Regardless of the validity of any or all of these definitions, this brief sample illustrates the range of perspectives employed in the identification of harassment and thereby suggests the problematic nature of supplying a comprehensive and consensual definition.

Returning to the areas of definitional agreement; i.e., that harassment is behavior of a sexual nature which is unwelcome, it is apparent that even these agreed upon guidelines may be insufficient for identification of harassment due to the complexity of the context of interaction. The problems of identification arise when these abstract areas of agreement are operationalized in terms of communicative behaviors between the harasser and the target. For instance, how does one identify a behavior which is sexual in nature? To answer this question one would have to consider socially construed meanings of the behaviors in light of sex role expectations and the possibility of multiple meanings for the same behavior. In the case of

[3]U.S. Office of Merit Systems Protection Board, Office of Review and Studies, "Rules of the Equal Employment Opportunity Commission," (Washington, D.C.: Bureau of National Affairs, 1981), pp. 13-14.

sexually harassing behaviors this distinction is often difficult. Furthermore, the target's perceived meaning for the behavior may not agree with the perpetrator's intent. Considering the second area of agreement, how does one identify a behavior as "unwelcome?" Common sense suggests that any subsequent answer would result from an investigation of the response of the target. In short, that the focus would have to be on the interaction between the communicators rather than on the behaviors or context alone. The following sections discuss the impact of sex role expectations, intent, and target response on the identification of sexually harassing incidents in terms of the difficulty of answering either of these questions.

Generally, sex role expectations in Western society dictate that men should behave in a dominant and controlling manner, while women should be nurturant and dependent. However, the influx of women into organizations and positions of power in this century has required women to eschew sex role stereotypes in order to meet expectations of competence in the work setting as Dr. Putnam discusses in the next chapter. The professional woman is caught in the tug-of-war between appropriately feminine and appropriately task oriented behavior expectations. This dilemma affects the propensity of female employees to employ traditionally masculine dominance behaviors. A study of dominance behaviors in organizational settings reported that male employees felt comfortable using both verbal and nonverbal dominance behaviors, although female employees felt they were behaving inappropriately when they employed the same behaviors.[4] In the instance of sexual harassment these sex role stereotypes are important when harassment is considered as dominance behavior.

Sexual harassment has been described as "a power game rather than a display of sexual interest."[5] Viewed in this way sexually harassing behaviors may be dominance behaviors

---

[4]Catherine Radecki and Joyce Jennings, "Sex as a Status Variable in Work Settings: Female and Male Reports of Dominance Behavior," *Journal of Applied Social Psychology*, 10 (1980), p. 71.

[5]Claire Safran, "Sexual Harassment: The View from the Top: The Joint Redbook-Harvard Business Review Report," *Redbook Magazine*, 156 (1981), p. 51.

that are interpreted in a sexual connotation. The behaviors themselves remain the same, and as some authors have suggested, may serve both purposes since dominance and intimacy behaviors are often interchangeable.[6] Possible multiplicity of meaning for the same behavior in combination with sex role expectations for organizational members may affect perceptions of situations that may be harassing and may dictate responses to harassment which are counterproductive.

The view of harassment as dominance behavior has contributed to the widely held opinion that harassment occurs primarily in superior-subordinate relationships. Many people assume that the situation cannot be considered harassment unless the perpetrator has control over the rewards or punishments for the target. The emphasis on unequal status relationships as the necessary context of harassment requires that people can and do distinguish between conventional status-related dominance behaviors and sexually harassing behaviors. Superiors in an organizational setting may frequently employ dominance behaviors as an expression of their elevated status. A woman subordinate working under a male superior must also consider the impact of sex role expectations on her superior's behavior. In such a context a single behavior could be explained as either a result of status differences, sex role expectations, sexual motivations or a combination of any or all factors. Obviously, simply stating that behavior of a sexual nature constitutes harassment is not sufficient in identifying harassing behaviors in these complex conditions.

The ambituity of "harassing" behaviors also affects the potential responses to harassment. If a woman subordinate feels harassed by a male superior she may be unwilling or unable to respond with behaviors which are considered socially inappropriate. Extremely negative reactions to such sexual advances may violate expectations for "feminine" behavior as well as expectations for appropriate "subordinate" behavior. Yet, if the target follows sex role and status-related expectations for behavior she may be unable to communicate effectively the unwelcome nature of these actions. Moreover, if the

[6]*Op. Cit.*, Radecki and Jennings, p. 82.

woman does not communicate her displeasure other organizational members may assume that she is accepting or even
appreciative of this type of attention. The female target of
harassment is placed in a situation of incurring the consequences of inappropriate role behavior or relinquishing peer
support in any attempt to curtail further harassment.

In addition to this already complex scenario an assessment
of the harassing nature of an interaction requires consideration of the motives or intent of the harasser. While not excusing
harassment in any form, it is nonetheless possible that a superior or co-worker may not realize that their behavior could be
considered harassment; especially in cases where the
"harasser" is behaving "appropriately" in terms of his understanding of sex or status related behaviors.

The Prevalence of Sexual Harassment

Even with the uncertainty involved in identifying sexual
harassment recent surveys indicate that organizational
members consider harassment a serious and prevalent
problem. The survey results reported in this section should be
received cautiously however. The consistently high amounts of
harassment reported are significant as indications of the magnitude of this problem, although the results of these surveys
are not completely generalizeable due to inconsistencies in the
definitions of harassment employed in the surveys and other
methodological shortcomings.

The Women's Section of the Human Affairs program at
Cornell University surveyed 155 working women at a conference on sexual harassment and related problems. 92% of these
women considered sexual harassment a serious problem as
one would expect from their participation in the conference.
However, compelling justification for their concern is evident
in the reports that 70% of these women had experienced some
form of harassment and that 56% of this latter group had
suffered physical harassment.[7] A study of 875 United Nations
employees, conducted in 1975, found that 49% of the women

[7]Terry L. Leap and Edmund R. Gray, "Corporate Responsibility in Cases of
Sexual Harassment," *Business Horizons*, 23 (1980), p. 58.

working at the United Nations reported experiencing sexual pressures on the job.[8] An exhaustive survey jointly conducted by the *Harvard Business Review* and *Redbook Magazine* in 1980 questioned thousands of subscribers and organizational employees. A vast majority of these respondents stated that sexual harassment was a serious problem in their work environment.[9]

Similar results have been obtained from surveys conducted in public sector organizations. In the fall of 1979, Sangamon State University researchers surveyed over 4,000 employees of the Illinois state government. 59% of the people surveyed reported having experienced one or more incidents of sexual harassment in their present place of employment.[10] The most comprehensive and methodologically sound survey available was conducted by the Federal Government's Merit System Protection Board Office of Review and Studies during the May 1978 to May 1980 time period. Responses from over 23,000 Office of Personnel Management employees revealed that at least 42% of female employees and 15% of male employees had been victims of sexual harassment during this two year period. The implications of this finding in terms of the quantity of people affected are staggering. As the report extrapolates, the survey results indicate that sexual harassment is a serious problem for approximately 294,000 female and 168,000 male federal government employees.[11]

Survey research and case studies supply information about variables that affect perceptions of sexual harassment incidents. An individual's perceptions of the severity of harassment or the recognition of harassment may depend upon their sex as well as the status of the "harasser."

Men and women perceive instances of harassment or potential harassment differently. Generally women are more sensitive than men to instances involving relatively ambiguous

[8]*Ibid.*, p. 58.

[9]Eliza G.C. Collins and Timothy B. Blodgett, "Some See It...Some Won't", *Harvard Business Review*, 59 (1981), p. 77.

[10]Michele Hoyman and Ronda Robinson, "Interpreting the New Sexual Harassment Guidelines," *Personnel Journal*, 59 (1980), p. 996.

[11]*Op. Cit.*, Merit Systems Protection Board, 1981, p. 33.

behaviors. Women are more likely than men to regard sexual innuendos, sexual references, sexual jokes, touching, and leering as harassing behaviors. In addition, women usually perceive the existence of a greater amount of sexual harassment than men. Except for extremely blatant sexual propositions the gender of the interpretor will probably affect the identification of a behavior or an interaction as sexually harassing.

The organizational status of the "harasser" affects perceptions of the existence and severity of harassment. Consistent with the view that harassment is generally restricted to superior-subordinate interactions survey research suggests that organizational members consider questionable behavior from a superior as more serious and threatening than equivalent behavior from a subordinate.[12] Since harassment is conceptually and in some cases definitionally identified in terms of the rewards or punishments associated with compliance or lack of compliance people tend to assume that control over resources increases the possibility of harassment.

These varying perceptions of potentially harassing situations may affect a woman's ability to deal effectively with harassing behavior. Irrespective of the organization there is a strong probability that higher status positions are disproportionately occupied by men. Therefore the professional woman may find little support from male peers who may not regard behaviors as harassing which the woman has interpreted as such. If harassment comes from a co-worker the victim may not be able to convince other organizational members that the situation demands their support since the consequences of harassment are not obvious in terms of occupational resources.

The prevalence of sexual harassment raises the issue of responses to harassment. Unfortunately, many tactics commonly employed by female victims of harassment may be partly responsible for the overwhelming incidence of this behavior. These responses may be a function of the time and place of harassment as well as the socially mandated possibilities for behavior. Severe sexual harassment often occurs in isolation, hidden from the view of other workers. In these cases

---

[12]*Op. Cit.*, Collins and Blodgett, p. 79.

women are placed in a "their-word-against-mine" situation. More subtle instances of harassment, such as touching or sexual innuendos, are more likely to occur in the presence of others. However, witnesses to such interactions may not regard the behaviors as harassing or as not serious enough to merit their support of the victim especially if the victim does not display overt displeasure.

As a result, the responses of many women faced with sexual harassment often appear passive, or at least, resigned. In the initial stages the overwhelming majority of women victims try to ignore the behaviors. This tactic is rarely effective in dissuading the harasser and may even goad the harasser into more severe actions.[13] A large percentage of women try to avoid further contact with the harasser. However, this is hardly a realistic alternative if the harasser is the woman's direct superior or an office mate. The usual ineffectiveness of passive responses can force the victim into a choice between quitting her job, sticking it out, or taking some type of formal action against the harasser. Unfortunately, many women choose the first alternative and quit, often without making any formal complaint against the harasser. Women who attempt to wait out the situation face the strong possibility of being punished for non-compliance with the sexual demands. One management consultant stated that she believes "more women are refused employment, are fired, or are forced to quit their jobs as a result of sexual demands and the consequences than of any other single cause."[14]

While outsiders may suggest that a blunt "no" is the appropriate alternative the immediate risk of unemployment, demotion, or reduced benefits in the workplace often discourages the victim from asserting their position. Even when this tactic is used there is the risk that the target may simply appear to be a more interesting challenge to the harasser.

Research concerning the prevalence of sexual harassment in organizations suggests that harassment is a major issue in

[13]Op. Cit., Farley, p. 22.
[14]Kathryn Thurston, "Sexual Harassment: An Organizational Perspective," Personnel Administrator, 25 (1980), p. 60.

need of action. Women who are victimized by harassing behavior seem to employ passive strategies which fail to deal effectively with this situation. Their responses may be limited due to expectations of their behavior which create a dilemma entailing violation of one or more norm sets in the organization. This vicious circle may be responsible for the high rates of reported harassment in survey research and definitely contributes to the individual and organizational consequences of harassment.

The Consequences of Sexual Harassment

The consequences of sexual harassment for the individual and the organization are extremely expensive in terms of either physical or financial well-being. Sexual harassment produces stress for the individual which often leads to what Backhouse and Cohen call the "sexual harassment syndrome." This syndrome, "caused by fending off unsolicited and offensive advances, causes tension, anxiety, frustration and anger."[15] The majority of sexual harassment victims experience emotional stress, physical illness and decreased performance capacity. The Merit System Protection Board Office of Review and Studies survey suggests some of the financial costs associated with harassment. They report that the physical and emotional stress suffered by the individual costs approximately five million dollars per year for the federal government employees alone. Many individual victims must personally bear the costs of physical and emotional illness caused by the harassment situation.

Organizationally the stress of sexual harassment may result in major expenditures from lost productivity and personnel functions needed to replace workers who choose to quit their jobs rather than endure the situation. Organizations suffer millions of dollars of loss each year in terms of decreased productivity resulting from sexual harassment stresses and concomitant absenteeism. Some sources estimate that the total

[15]Constance Backhouse and Leah Cohen, The Secret Oppression: The Sexual Harassment of Working Women (Toronto, Canada: MacMillan 1978), p. 45.

turnover costs in replacing the victims who quit is in excess of a billion dollars annually.[16]

The consequences of sexual harassment; particularly turnover, absenteeism, and decreased performance, affect a vast array of personnel activities in the organization. Yet, remedies for this problem, if they exist at all, are usually only reactive rather than proactive. In essence, the organization attempts to deal with the effects of harassment after the fact instead of working to prevent harassment in the work place. Recent litigation concerning the possibility of holding the employer financially liable for the harassing behaviors of its employees is stimulating organizations to develop more proactive responses to the harassment problem. This litigation also results in significant hazards for the organizations should they fail in their protection of all employees from such discriminatory behavior.

Although victims of sexual harassment may seek redress through criminal or civil tort legal proceedings, the primary avenue of recourse has been civil litigation under Title VII. Title VII of the Civil Rights Act of 1964, as amended by the Equal Employment Opportunity Act of 1972, prohibits sex discrimination in any term, condition, or privilege of employment.[17] In several recent court decisions sexual harassment has been identified as a form of sexual discrimination.[18]

Determination of employer liability means that the employer is held responsible for the harassing actions of superviosry as well as non-supervisory personnel. Only a few cases have resulted in decisions against the employer. All of these cases involved a situation of male superior and female subordinate harassment.

Earlier cases such as *Barnes v. Costle*, and *Tomkins v. Public Service Electric and Gas Co.*, ruled against the employer but exempted the employer from liability if prompt remedial action was taken. A different logic was used in the *Miller v. Bank of*

---

[16]*Op. Cit.*. Merit Systems Protection Board, 1981, p. 76.
[17]Catherine MacKinnon, *Sexual Harassment of Working Women* (New Haven, Connecticut: Yale University Press, 1979), p. 6.
[18]*Ibid.*, pp. 57-100.

America case in which the court held that the employer was liable even if the company had a policy prohibiting sexual harassment and even when the victim did not normally notify the employer of the situation. Two decisins have focused on the employer's responsibility for investigating incidents of harassment. *Munford v. James T. Barnes and Co.* and *Bundy v. Jackson* found the employer liable if they failed to investigate complaints of sexual harassment.

Although there are too few cases to establish a strong precedent in the area of employer liability the existing decisions suggest that an employer may be held responsible for an employee's harassing behavior if it can be shown that the harassment was done with management's knowledge, or if management had a chance to rectify the situation and did not. Future cases will undoubtedly qualify the conditions which determine employer liability. Appeal actions on cases reported or already litigated may redefine the criteria discussed in these instances. Readers who are interested in a thorough review of the legal actions taken in cases of sexual harassment are urged to examine the work of Catherine MacKinnon[19] who has chronicled the relevant decisions and accompanying logic of the decisions through the late 1970s.

The threat of employer liability decisions entails several costs to the organization. Decisions against the employer may force the organization to provide back pay to the grievant, to assume the victim's legal expenses, and possibly to pay further damages to the victim. The organization also suffers in terms of public image. It is important to remember that these costs are in addition to productivity losses and personnel costs which the organization may have already incurred.

In addition, the EEOC Guidelines on Sexual Harassment take a strong position in favor of victims of harassment. The Guidelines detail specific policies and actions required of employers including: "Affirmatively raising the subject of sexual harassment, expressing strong disapproval, informing all employees of their Title VII rights, developing investigation procedures, developing appropriate sanctions and disciplinary channels,

---

[19]*Ibid.*

and developing methods to sensitize all employees to this problem."[20] Failure to comply with the Guidelines may critically affect sexual harassment litigation and may result in loss of federal contracts depending upon the severity of the infractions. The strength of the Guidelines is dependent upon changes in the Guidelines and the allocation of manpower to enforce-these provisions. Therefore, victims of harassment as well as organizations need to keep abreast of changes in the political and legal decisions concerning this enforcement.

Women need to be mindful of their options if they are or have been victims of sexual harassment. In unionized organizations the grievance procedure may provide some remedies for victims of harassment. If the organization has a formal policy against sexual harassment the victim may find assistance through the personnel department disciplinary procedures or through recourse to top management. Especially if the organization has declared its position publicly, it may be more willing to take actions to protect the interests of the victim.

Combatting Sexual Harassment

There are several actions which may prove effective in dealing with sexual harassment. Primarily, the woman being harassed must take action to let the harasser and other workers know that this behavior is offensive and unwelcome. These actions may begin with a statement to the harasser that a specific behavior is bothersome and should be discontinued. Often an employee can confront the harasser by listing the specific behaviors and instances she regards as harassing in as much detail as possible. If this tactic fails the victim may write a letter concerning the problem and the fact that initial confrontation with the harasser was ineffective in gaining his or her cooperation. The letter should be as comprehensive as possible, listing the names and dates of harassment incidents as well as the confrontation.[21] The letter should be sent to the

---

[20]Grace Mastalli, "The Legal Context," *Harvard Business Review,* 59 (1981), p. 94.

[21]Mary P. Rowe, "Dealing with Sexual Harassment," *Harvard Business Review,* 59 (1981), p. 45.

personnel department, to the harasser's direct superior, and to the harasser. In conjunction, any victim of sexual harassment should try to get witnesses who will testify on his or her behalf. This may prove crucial to the success of remedial actions. Finally, all organizational members should inform themselves about their legal rights in a sexual harassment situation.

Victims of harassment can attempt to gain support by talking with co-workers, by letting others know what is going on in incidents of harassment which occur in isolation, or by calling attention to behaviors which have been observed by others. By creating this awareness of potential harassment the woman may persuade other workers to take individual action as well. The chances are that other people in the same work environment have experienced similar pressures or have witnessed the situation between the victim and the harasser. If so, an effective peer support system may be the most expedient informal remedy available to the victim.

The organization can and should institute proactive personnel policies to deal with sexual harassment in the workplace. Proactive policies necessary for compliance with the EEOC Guidelines involve four activities: 1) issuing a statement of corporate policy on sexual harassment; 2) developing training programs for superiors and subordinates; 3) establishing adequate investigation procedures for such cases; and 4) developing and utilizing quick and effective methods of disciplinary action.

The issuance of a corporate policy statement concerning sexual harassment clarifies the organization's position and may prevent questionable behavior. Such policy statements also supply employees with an indication of the support that they can expect to receive from the organization if such a problem arises.

Training programs for supervisors, as well as orientation programs for new employees should include instructions for recognizing sexual harassment or potentially harassing behaviors, discussions of internal and external sanctions, and explanation of avenues of redress for victims of harassment. Personnel managers can utilize in-house communication to update employees on recent legal and corporate actions concerning sexual harassment.

The establishment of an investigation procedure is critical in light of decisions in the area of employer liability. This procedure should be available to all employees, preferably allowing for maximum confidentiality. Such procedures may conflict with existing grievance procedures in unionized companies; therefore conciliation between the systems may be necessary. The steps in the investigation procedure and the actions taken as a result of an investigation need to be carefully documented for employee and employer protection in the case of further litigation. A truly proactive policy would include a review of performance appraisal and internal staffing decisions which may signal repetitive use of loopholes in the performance documentation that could affect litigation results. If such patterns can be determined at an early stage action can be taken to preclude the possibility of harassment.

Finally, and most importantly, the organization must annouce and act upon sanctions detailed in the disciplinary procedure. If a union represents employees the employer must work cooperatively with the union to insure acceptance of the sanctions. These actions, if warranted, should be swiftly and impartially enforced according to the announced policy of the organization.

It would be pleasant to conclude that the recent interest in the problem of sexual harassment signifies a dramatic shift in the public and organizational attitudes toward this problem. It is hopeful that more people seem to be aware of the magnitude of the problem and its consequences. Yet, an effective campaign against sexual harassment has only begun. Its success depends upon the willingness of organizational members to invest and inform themselves for their own protection. By working with interested and concerned management, organizational members may be able to bring this effort to fruition.

Lady You're Trapped:
Breaking Out of Conflict Cycles

Linda L. Putnam

Whether we realize it or not, women in organizations are frequently trapped. No matter what situation they encounter or which individual they talk with, they may face the barrier of being "damned if you do and damned if you don't." This vulnerability for getting boxed-into situations stems, in part, from the precarious role of women in organizations. Women function as representatives of their sex while simultaneously trying to liberate themselves from the negative aspects of their stereotype. As aspiring executives they are told to behave assertively and independently while being criticized for becoming paradies of men. When a woman takes charge of a situation and begins to issue orders, she is viewed as the "bitch" who abandoned her role as the nurturant leader. When a woman excels in her profession, she is perceived as "pushy and competitive," traits that are not only unbecoming to the feminine species but also threatening to men. In many organizational circumstances, it appears that women just can't win.

While it is easy to become discouraged with such dilemmas and to withdraw from the scene, it is a better tactic to recognize and cope with the situation. Being trapped is a form of a "double bind." Even though a woman experiences the sensation of "damned if you do and damned if you don't," she still has a choice. Although that choice is frequently between two undesirable actions, a choice exists and can be managed without severe loss of credibility. But even before a woman feels trapped, she participates, usually unconsciously, in the events

39

that lead to the "double bind." Hence, a second way of coping with organizational dilemmas is to recognize the evolution of a "double bind" and to respond to the symptoms rather than to the outcome of being trapped. What are the symbols of "double binds?" What types of messages lead a person into traps? How are "double binds" created by the way we infer meanings to events? How are these patterns related to the management of conflict? Symptoms of the "double bind" first appear in contradictory messages. This paper describes the way contradictory messages lead to "double binds." In addition, it discusses why women in organizations are victimized by "double binds" and what women can do to recognize and manage the symptoms of these conflict cycles.

Contradictory Messages and Conflict Cycles

Contradictions, while not always intentional, frequently appear in our interactions with others. On the one hand we acknowledge and readily accept the fact that people change their minds, but on the other hand we measure predictability of human behavior with the yardstick of consistency. Hence, if a supervisor comments that she has plenty of time to discuss a problem while she simultaneously fidgits and looks at her watch, we draw the conclusion that the verbal and nonverbal messages are contradictory. The supervisor is saying on the verbal level that she is available and willing to talk with us but on the nonverbal level she projects a feeling of being rushed and nervous. Even though the supervisor may not be aware of her contradictory cues, the subordinate must take into account both the verbal and the nonverbal messages. The subordinate must either accept one message and ignore the inconsistency or reconcile the contradiction. For example, the subordinate could infer that the supervisor is busy and would rather not talk. Therefore, the supervisor's verbal response is a sign of politeness. In this instance, the subordinate would arrange to discuss the problem at another time. Or the subordinate might attribute the superior's nonverbal message to a general state of anxiety. In this case, the subordinate would ignore the nonverbal message and heed the verbal cue.

A third but less likely response is to expose the contradiction. Specifically, the subordinate might remark, "While you seem to be free right now, I see you are looking at your watch. Do you have an impending appointment?" Of course, the supervisor can deny the contradicton and continue to emit an inconsistent message. Regardless of the response, the resultant interaction between the supervisor and subordinate is affected by *the perception* of a contradictory message. A contradiction, in this sense, refers to two or more messages with opposite meanings; hence both messages cannot be simultaneously correct. It is illogical to infer that the supervisor in the previous example wants to talk with the subordinate about his or her problem while not wanting to talk with this person. The two behaviors are logically inconsistent. Contradictory messages, however, evolve from the way that we tie observed behaviors to verbal messages. These linkages are *inferences* or *interpretations* of meaning for events. Our interpretations, however, may not parallel what actually happened or what the other person intended to say. But once we see two messages as contradictory, this perception influences future communication. In effect, meanings that we attribute to perceived contradictions guide the way that we initiate and respond to future interactions with this person.

Since we derive meanings in human interaction from multiple levels of communication, it is possible for contradictions to exist between two verbal messages as well as between verbal and nonverbal levels. For instance, a supervisor might assign an employee a particular task and then reprimand·him for assuming the responsibilities that the supervisor assigned. While this example sounds absurd, a full story might reveal that the supervisor's boss disapproves of this assignment. When the boss complains, the supervisor saves face by reprimanding the subordinate for spending time on the project. The supervisor, in this instance, employs contradictory verbal messages to avoid a confrontation with his or her boss and to save face with his or her subordinate. The subordinate, however, sees only the contradictory request and remains baffled and frustrated by the mixed message. If the subordinate exposes the contradiction, the supervisor can claim that the employee misunderstood his or her original message or that the request was only a suggestion, not a specific assignment.

You may be thinking that contradictory messages are rather commonplace in organizational settings. Indeed they are, particularly if we consider that coordinating a large organization involves simultaneous communication among many individuals. It is not unusual to receive a message from one person and an opposite one from another employee. This type of communication occurs daily in the lives of most organizational members. Although contradictions between people arouse concern, these inconsistencies are usually managed by getting individuals together to reconcile their incongruent requests.

Contradictions that emanate from the same person, however, particularly a supervisor or a member of upper management, are particularly perplexing for a number of reasons. First, they cross status boundaries in organizations. There is an unwritten protocol that prohibits us from accusing another person of using contradictory messages. Such an accusation implies that the other person's communication is inadequate or that the other person is deceiving us in some way. Hence, in any situation it is difficult to challenge the use of a contradictory message. But when the other person is your supervisor, the risk of challenging a contradiction is even greater, particularly since it is easy for the accused to deny such incongruencies. In effect, status differences between superior and subordinate intensify the problem of responding to contradictory messages.

Secondly, subordinates rely on supervisors for upward mobility and for information about the organization. This dependency is even more pronounced for women in organizations than it is for men. Females report that meetings with their supervisors and contacts with upper management directly contribute to company advancements. Men, in contrast, attribute their promotions to their own achievements or to their training. Research has shown that women, who advance in traditional masculine organizations, must break through a sex-structured filtering system, one protected by political alliances and connections with managerial personnel. Since women depend on their supervisors for upward contacts in the organization, they take greater risks when they confront their supervisors than do their male counterparts.

A third reason that a supervisor's contradictory messages

are perplexing is that most subordinates genuinely want to abide by the directions of their superior. That is, subordinates would like to give their supervisors the benefit of the doubt. When a contradictory message occurs, the subordinate attributes it to a communication breakdown. But if the contradiction persists, the subordinate begins to question the motives of the supervisor.

This process of imputing motives for incongruent messages leads to what is known as a conflict cycle or a double bind. A conflict cycle is a self-perpetuating circle of cause-effect behaviors. All of us have heard the case of the alcoholic husband who contends that he drinks because his wife is an excessive nagger. His wife, of course, reminds him that she would not nag him if he would quit drinking. Both are caught in a conflict cycle where one person's behavior serves as the cause for the other person's response. She argues, "I would not be a nagger if you were not a drinker." He contends, "I would not be a drinker if you had never nagged me." A conflict cycle, then, argues which came first, the chicken or the egg. Following this style of argument perpetuates this cycle and leads the participants into a predictable 'rut.' Sometimes this routine takes the form of a "double bind," the feeling of being "damned if you do and damned if you don't."

For example, a conflict cycle in an organization occurred when a recently promoted supervisor, Michael, gathered his subordinates for a strategy session. During the session Michael and his subordinates plotted job responsibilities, delegated tasks, and worked in a participatory manner. In fact, Michael explicitly stated that he saw his role as primarily a facilitator for the workers. He encouraged his subordinates to participate in the work process and in the decision-making aspects of his job. But when the work began to pile up and the pressure was on, the supervisor arrived early and stayed after hours to complete the tasks he had delegated to his workers. Gradually, the employees had less and less to do. They responded with passivity and general apathy toward their jobs. Michael gave a contradictory message of "Participate by not doing anything." On the verbal level he urged employees to get involved, but on the nonverbal level he discouraged their participation by indicating that he did not trust them to do the job well. In truth,

Michael just couldn't turn loose of the day-to-day operations of the work unit. He saw himself as a dedicated participatory manager, but he failed to realize that his close supervision was inconsistent with his verbal request, "to participate in the work process."

The conflict cycle ensued when Michael used his subordinates' reactions as evidence for his own behavior. He evaluated his subordinates as lazy and apathetic. He cited instances of their passivity and their lack of enthusiasm for the work. While one employee psychologically withdrew, the other responded with physical avoidance in the form of tardiness and absenteeism. The more his subordinate withdrew, the more Michael tried to compensate for employee laziness by working harder. When asked why he was such a zealot about his work, Michael responded that his employees left him no choice. As the cycle began to snowball, Michael approached his manager and received permission to have one employee transferred to another department and to have the other one severely reprimanded for poor job performance.

The sad part of this story was the failure of the participants to recognize the contradictory message, conflict cycles, and double bind. The subordinates ignored the command "to participate" and accepted the "by not doing anything" portion of Michael's contradictory message. Rather than confront Michael, they blamed him for their predicament and felt trapped by their own inactivity. Michael, in turn, perpetuated the conflict cycle by blaming his subordinates for his own behavior. But the blame did not lie in the people or the situation. Rather it resided in the process of their communication. Because there was a kernel of truth to both sides of this story, the cycle could not be broken with a circular cause-effect argument. The real issue was not who caused the dilemma, but whether either party had the ability to expose it and to accept both sides of the story. The employees were correct in their accusation about their workaholic supervisor and Michael was accurate in his observation about his apathetic workers. Neither party, however, recognized that a conflict cycle was in effect.

Another specific instance of a vicious cycle was a supervisor who advised his female subordinate to budget her time wisely and to take on only those additional responsibilities that would lead to her career advancement. Then he asked her to undertake trivial, mundane projects that would contribute only a modicum to her promotion. The supervisor gave the message, "Think of your career advancement first while you devote your time to my special projects." Other examples of contradictory messages are: "Make your own decisions by checking to see what I want you to do;" "Be assertive by not confronting me," and "Be competent and firm but don't appear threatening to anyone."

Women as Victims of Conflict Cycles

Women in organizations are easily victimized by conflict cycles and double binds. First, women are already entrapped in society's stereotypes for traditional feminine behavior. Our culture typically depicts women as emotional, passive, dependent, nurtural, intuitive, and submissive. The successful leader in our society is viewed as a person who is aggressive, forceful, competitive, achievement-oriented, self-confident, and independent. These are personality traits that typically characterize males in our society. A woman who aspires to be a manager frequently faces a culturally-defined double bind. If she behaves like an effective leader, she is condemned for being unfeminine. If she displays the culturally-defined traits of a woman, she is deemed unfit for a managerial position. To function within this prescribed double bind, a woman must find the "happy medium" between masculine and feminine roles. But males who are resentful or skeptical about a female manager may use subtle contradictory cues to invoke this double bind.

Robert Schrank, in his story of "Two Women, Three Men on a Raft," provides an excellent example of this type of conflict cycle.[1] The chronicle begins in a survival training camp sponsored by Outward Bound. The staff trainers emphasize the perils of river running and the imminent dangers that lurk in

---

[1] Robert Schrank, "Two Women and Three Men on a Raft," *Harvard Business Review*, 55 (1977), 100-108.

the wilderness beyond the camp. The participants are assigned
to teams of four and five members to a raft. Each team is
responsible for survival during the seven days of running the
Rogue River. On Schrank's raft are three men and two women,
all in their mid-fifties. Both women are professionals, one a
president of a small fund-raising organization and the other a
first-line supervisor. One of the males is a successful lawyer,
the other is a teacher, and the third, a staff specialist for a
large foundation.

Under the requirements of the Outward Bound program,
each person must guide the raft during the trip. The contradictory message starts when one woman takes the helm and
begins to complain of getting tired. When she alludes to her
apprehensions about maneuvering the raft, the men chime in,
"This is nothing. You should canoe the St. John." Thus, the men
put on a patriarchal air and advise the women about the
proper procedures for using the helm. When one of the 'girls'
cries, "I can't do it," a male colleague pauses for a moment,
sighs, then gives her a fatherly, "You're doing just fine. You
can do it." But his voice tone and evasive eye contact shouts,
"When is she going to give up!!!" Through contradictory
messages, the women are subtly trapped in a conflict cycle.
These messages reinforce self-doubts and contribute to a self-
fulfilling prophecy of failure. This experience, in Schrank's
opinion, parallels male response to female leadership in corporate settings. Through fears of relinquishing power, males
unconsciously sabotage the leadership efforts of women. When
women get trapped in conflict cycles, it's difficult for them to
win.

A second way that women are easily victimized by conflict
cycles stems from the dualistic roles of token and professional.
As a representative of her sex, a woman must undertake the
role of a token in addition to the duties of her position. A token
represents the organization in a variety of endeavors. She is
subject to the pleas: "We need a woman on this committee"
and "Look over this document on promotion and tell me how it
affects minorities" and "Help us recruit more competent
women in the organization." These appeals underscore the importance of a woman's role while simultaneously reminding
her that she is a token. In many instances this token status

works for the advancement of women, but it can also hinder a woman's efforts. The term "woman" becomes synonymous with "affirmative action candidate"; hence her accomplishments are frequently evaluated within this category. She hears statements like, "Not a bad job for an affirmative action candidate" and "I've promoted three affirmative action candidates. They never make the grade," and "Affirmative action candidates don't automatically get promoted." Thus, in addition to struggling with cultural stereotypes, women must also combat the conflict cycles associated with their status as tokens.

A final reason why women are frequently victimized by conflict cycles stems from male-female approaches to the management of organizational conflicts. People typically respond to contradictory messages in ways that help manage the conflict. Some people withdraw, either psychologically or physically, through silence, absenteeism, or superficial interaction. Others react by challenging one level of the contradiction. This response sometimes leads to the cause-effect cycle that we see with the alcoholic husband and the nagging wife. Others deny the situation by pretending it isn't happening to them. This type of withdrawal can lead to a feeling of being paralyzed in the situation.

Males and females differ in their perceptions of and approaches to the management of organizational conflicts. These differences are likely to affect the way men and women respond to contradictory messages. Even though traditional stereotypes depict men as competitive and women as cooperative, current research reveals a more complex picture of male-female conflict behavior. Specifically, the sex of the other person influences an individual's approach to conflict situations. Naturally, if we like the other person, we are more willing to collaborate on a solution than we are if we dislike them. This finding is consistent for same-sex and opposite-sex relationships. Two males, however, are less likely to negotiate an equitable settlement than are two females. Two males in a conflict typically employ bargaining techniques, logical arguments, and anger to manage the situation. In contrast, two females in a conflict situation focus on understanding each other's feelings. Thus, there appear to be general differences in male-female styles of managing conflict. These style differences, however, do not necessarily mean that women select cooperative outcomes. In fact, in laboratory investigations of bargaining behavior, an equal number of studies show that men are more cooperative than women.

Research in organizational settings reveals that females prefer to handle conflicts by smoothing over difficulties, by playing down differences, and by emphasizing similarities. Males, in contrast, report a negative reaction to smoothing as a form of conflict management, particularly when their supervisor uses this mode to resolve disagreements. Both males and females react favorably to the use of compromise as a form of conflict management. Another study reveals differences in the sex-role composition of supervisor-subordinate conflicts. Disagreements are more likely to be discussed openly if the supervisor is a woman. Both male and female subordinates who report to female supervisors frequently confront her about disagreements whereas those who report to a male supervisor typically withdraw from conflict situations. In general, when the supervisor is a male, conflict is not easy to handle. Differences in male-female styles of conflict management and difficulties in confronting male supervisors suggest that withdrawal is a common response to contradictory messages. Moreover, when the conflict centers on a woman's role, it is even harder to confront a male supervisor about contradictory cues.

Effective Management of Conflict Cycles

Even though withdrawal is a natural reaction to a conflict cycle, it is not necessarily the most effective response. Other alternatives for managing conflict fall into the categories of prevention and resolution. Of course, the most desirable alternative is to prevent the escalation of conflict cycles. Listed below are some guidelines to help avoid double binds.

1. Develop skills in process analysis by viewing organizations as sets of tightly integrated events. This process approach allows a person to rise above specific behaviors, to see the whole picture, and to avoid the pitfalls of "cause-effect" or "either-or" ways of thinking. This perspective encourages a

person to reflect upon past conversations and to recap events that led to problems. A process view also helps an individual uncover contradictory messages before they develop into conflict cycles. When someone becomes a victim of contradictory messages, his or her reflex response is to blame the other person or to suspect his or her motives. If both people function in a fault-finding manner, both will perpetuate the cycle by subtly communicating these suspicions.

2. Reflect a consistent image of self-confidence, especially in situations where a person can be easily trapped. In the example of three men and two women on a raft, the act of sharing self-doubts made the women vulnerable to conflict cycles. In effect, they provided the stimuli for the contradictory message. While all of us have doubts about our own abilities, we should share these apprehensions with members of support groups rather than with supervisors and peers. An air of self-confidence can dispell stereotypic assumptions that lead to contradictory messages. In essence, women professionals should reflect a consistent image of self-confidence and avoid giving contradictory cues about their own behaviors.

3. Improve skills in confrontation and bargaining. Women should develop their abilities to confront issues directly and to negotiate favorable settlements. In developing these skills, women should expand their level of tolerance for the exchange of attack-defend arguments. Women must hold to their positions while allowing others to state their opinions and argue defensively. When an attack-defend argument leads to a compromise or settlement, women should avoid holding grudges and harboring emotional resentment toward other participants. One rule of thumb in bargaining is to ask for more than you are willing to accept. Because women tend to underestimate their worth or their positions, this rule of thumb is particularly applicable to female bargaining behavior. An ability to confront directly and to bargain for an equitable settlement aids in solving problems and in reducing opportunities for contradictory messages to emerge.

4. Manage the public presentation of winning and losing conflicts. Public visibility of conflict victories advertises a sudden power shift. This shift can build resentment among the losers and can lead to the intentional use of contradictory messages and conflict cycles. Women function most effectively in public conflicts by using peers as buffers or as lieutenants for their position. Also, disagreements with peers or supervisors are managed more effectively in an interpersonal setting than in a public meeting.

These guidelines represent preventative measures against the escalation of conflict cycles. But women do not always have control over the development of these dilemmas. When a woman recognizes that she is getting trapped in a conflict cycle, she can take action to break the spiral. Timing is of utmost importance in reacting to an existing cycle. The sooner one notices a conflict cycle, the easier it is to manage it. Once a cycle persists to the point of becoming a reality for both participants, it is very difficult to break the pattern without intervention from a neutral third person. In the early stages of a conflict cycle, there are several ways to break the pattern. First, an individual can expose the contradiction by talking about the double message. This type of confrontation, however, must be handled very judiciously and must be initiated in the early stages of the cycle. Specifically, a person must expose the contradiction without any indication of blame or any tendency to impute motives. To break the cycle a person must discuss the process rather than the cause of the situation. Hence, each individual should acknowledge his or her role in contributing to the dilemma in a concerned supportive manner. If a supervisor feels insecure or threatened by this confrontation, he or she may deny the contradiction while continuing to communicate with double messages. In this instance, talking about the contradition will **not** break the cycle.

A second way to break a conflict cycle is to alter the cause-effect thinking that forms the essence of this pattern. For example, in the contradictory message, "Be assertive by not confronting me," the causal link between these behaviors follows this pattern: assertive behaviors lead to confrontation with the supervisor which, in turn, threatens supervisor and influences his message, "Be assertive by not confronting me."

The diagram below illustrates this cycle.

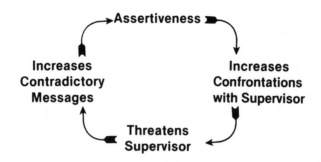

Notice that a line connects the supervisor's contradictory message and continued assertive behaviors of the woman. In effect, the cycle is sustained by accepting the "Be assertive" portion of the message and ignoring the second portion, "by not confronting me." This cycle can be broken in two ways: (1) changing perceptions about the links between these behaviors, (2) adding new behaviors that sever the cause-effect links in the existing spiral.

The woman could attempt to convince her boss that her assertiveness enhances his achievement. She could try to reduce his feelings of insecurity by demonstrating that his effectiveness as a supervisor is enhanced by her assertiveness. This strategy breaks the conflict cycle by making her assertiveness contribute to his effective job performance. This change should reduce his use of contradictory messages. In addition to modifying perceptions about the links between behaviors, the subordinate could add other explanations that are not included in the conflict cycle. For instance, she could show a connection between her assertiveness and her dedication to the company. Assertiveness, then, is defined as a positive factor that symbolizes her identification with the organization. She could show that her commitment to the organization is an outgrowth of his influence; hence her assertiveness enhances his influence in the organization.

While these strategies appear contrived, effective communicators develop skills in reframing experiences. This reframing changes the way people think about situations and prevents them from getting trapped in ruts. Some people readily develop the skills to reframe situations and to promote effective problem solving. Reframing experiences breaks the conflict cycle by creating new interpretations of events. When reframing is handled effectively, it is usually more successful in breaking conflict cycles than simply exposing the contradictory message.

A third way to break conflict cycles is to seek the input of a neutral third party. Deep-seated conflict cycles engender feelings of distrust between participants. A third person who is known and trusted by both parties can intervene and help reframe the situation. Sometimes simply talking with a neutral third person can help an individual interpret events differently. The third party can add plausible explanations for why the contradiction occurred and can suggest alternatives for managing a·conflict cycle. However, some risk is involved in consulting a third party. He or she could mismanage the intervention or could betray the confidence of the person who feels trapped; thus the choice of a neutral person is a critical decision.

Not all contradictory messages merit the time and energy for this type of conflict management. Even though withdrawal fails to break the conflict cycle, conflicts that occur infrequently or are too low in importance are often handled this way. If the contradictory message occurs between people who rarely interact with each other, then avoidance may be the best strategy for managing the conflict. It is easier to withdraw from a conflict cycle than it is to spend considerable time and emotional energy trying to break the spiral. In effect, we should not waste our energies on conflict cycles that are insignificant.

This paper addresses a prevalent and perplexing problem in organizational behavior — the evolution and effective management of conflict cycles. These cycles emerge from contradictory messages that get locked into cause-effect spirals. These cycles are particularly troublesome to women who are already trapped in society's double binds and in their roles as organizational tokens. Some conflict cycles can be prevented by improving our bargaining skills and by employing a process approach to organizational events. In circumstances where the emergence of conflict cycles are beyond our control, women can break these cycles by reframing interpretations of events and by seeking the advice or the intervention of a third party.

In his book, *The Social Psychology of Organizing,* Karl Weick points out that "most managers get into trouble because they forget to think in circles."[2] Once we realize that organizational events occur through interrelated behaviors, we understand the truth of this statement. In order to manage conflict cycles effectively, we must abandon our habits of thinking in simple cause-effect relationships and adopt a new way of analyzing organizational event. This new approach is to think in circles. If we reframe experiences by creating constructive interpretations for events, we avoid blaming others for contradictory messages and conflict cycles.

[2]Karl E. Weick, *The Social Psychology of Organizaing,* 2nd ed. (Reading, Massachusetts: Addison-Wesley Co., 1979), p. 86.

Women in Organizations: The Impact of Law

Lawrence Baum

In the past two decades the legal status of women in organizations has changed fundamentally. For the first time women who are students and employees have gained significant legal protections against sex discrimination.

This chapter is concerned with the impact of that legal change. To what extent has the situation of women in organizations actually improved as a result of the law? Do legal protections provide real protections for the woman who has suffered from discrimination? I will try to provide partial answers to these complicated questions by putting the laws against sex discrimination in a broader context.

The first section of the chapter will discuss changes in the law of sex discrimination as part of a general change in the legal status of students and employees. The chapter then will examine the impact of legal protections for women as one issue involving the effect of law in practice.

I

For most of American history the law allowed businesses and schools to conduct their internal affairs pretty much as their leaders saw fit. The treatment of employees and of students was at the discretion of those who stood above them in the organizational hierarchy, and they had little legal recourse if they felt that they had been treated unfairly.

For employees, the clearest expression of this general rule

was the legal doctrine that an employer could dismiss an employee at will. Unless an employee had specific contractual rights to continued employment, no protection of that employment existed. As one court stated the doctrine, employers "may dismiss their employees at will...for good cause, for no cause, or even for cause morally wrong, without being thereby guilty of legal wrong."[1] Employers had the same prerogatives in regard to the treatment of employees on the job, including the setting of pay and working conditions.

The legal status of students was similar to that of employees. Even at the college level students held few legal rights, as the courts formulated a set of doctrines to justify upholding the decisions of college authorities. One was the *in loco parentis* doctrine, under which college officials were treated as substitutes for parents. In this status they obtained some of the power that parents have to control their children. Another doctrine held that enrollment in a university was a privilege rather than a right, so that a student could not complain that a dismissal had been unjust. Judges' general willingness to allow arbitrary action by colleges is illustrated by a 1928 case in which a New York court upheld the dismissal of a Syracuse University student for the apparent offense of failing to be a "typical Syracuse girl."[2]

Both men and women lacked significant legal protection as students and employees. But this powerlessness had a more serious effect on women. Along with the arbitrary treatment that both sexes might face, women also had to cope with pervasive patterns of discrimination based on sex. In education, women were excluded from certain classes, programs, and even whole schools. In employment, women often were refused jobs, relegated to low-level jobs, or paid lower wages based on their sex.

The women who suffered from that discrimination had very little legal recourse. Indeed, American law itself was permeated with provisions that treated women and men differently, and the law also provided some support for sex discrimination

---

[1]*Payne v. Western & A.R.R.*, 81 Tenn. 507, §19-20 (1884).
[2]*Anthony v. Syracuse University*, 231 N.Y.S. 435 (App. Div. 1928).

by private organizations. A good example is the "protective" legislation of the early 20th century, which restricted women's employment opportunities by excluding them from some jobs or limiting the hours that they could work.[3] It should be noted as well that government-run schools and government employers were not substantially more dedicated to sexual equality than were their counterparts in the private sector.

Because there were no legal prohibitions against discrimination, organizations that treated women differently from men could be quite open about their practices. In 1922, for instance, the dean of the Columbia University Law School refused to open the law school to women. His rationale for a policy not to admit women was, "We don't because we don't."[4] As late as 1960 a survey of employers by the National Office Managers Association reportedly found that one-third openly admitted systematic wage discrimination against women.[5]

The discrimination against women that occurred in education and employment had a fundamental impact on the roles and status of women. In the aggregate, the various forms of sex discrimination in these sectors explain at least a large share of the substantial gap between the income of women and that of men.[6] More subtle but no less important was the impact of discrimination on women's opportunities for self-fulfillment through schooling and work. By accepting and encouraging distinctions between the sexes, the law was in part responsible for these effects of organizational discrimination.

Congress and the courts gradually have eroded the tradi-

[3]Whether these laws actually were intended to hurt women's employment status rather than to protect women from arduous conditions in employment is debated, and the motives may have been mixed. On the "protective" laws generally, see Barbara Babcock, Ann E. Freedman, Eleanor Holmes Norton, and Susan C. Ross, *Sex Discrimination and the Law* (Boston: Little, Brown, 1975), pp. 23-53, 268-287.

[4]The dean was Harlan Fiske Stone, later chief justice of the U.S. Supreme Court. Cynthia Fuchs Epstein, *Women in Law* (New York: Basic Books, 1981)., p. 51.

[5]Caroline Bird, *Born Female*, rev. ed. (New York: David McKay, 1970), p. 74.

[6]See Isabel V. Sawhill, "The Economics of Discrimination Against Women: Some New Findings," *Journal of Human Resources*, 8 (Summer, 1973), 383-394.

tional autonomy of organizations under the law. In the 1930s Congress adopted a series of laws that placed some limits on employers' setting of wages and responses to union organizing efforts. In the 1960s and 1970s Congress established a series of protections for both employees and students, ranging from prohibitions against racial discrimination to safeguards for student privacy. Increasingly the courts also have ruled that people within organizations hold some legal rights. For instance, several courts now have decided that students threatened with dismissal are entitled to procedural safeguards.

The extent of the change that has occurred should not be exaggerated. The legal rights of people within organizations remain limited in some important ways. This is particularly true of employees in private firms and students in private schools, to whom constitutional protections of civil liberties generally do not apply. A few years ago the owner of a football team reportedly announced that "Freedom of speech isn't carte blanche when you're taking someone's money;"[7] at least as a matter of law in the private sector, his statement was largely correct. At the same time, the changes that have occurred are significant in their implications. No longer are people in organizations powerless under the law.

This change in the legal position of organizations eventually reached the issue of sex discrimination. Just as the law has limited the prerogatives of organizations in other respects, it now limits differences in the treatment of the sexes in both employment and education. The most important part of this change had been the adoption by Congress and the president of four laws to attack discrimination in organizations.

1. The Equal Pay Act of 1963 amended the minimum wage law to prohibit discrimination in wages by sex, under a general "equal pay for equal work" provision. Under the Act an employer who is found guilty of discrimination may be required to equalize wages and to provide back pay to com-

---

[7]Red Smith, "Grass on Buckwheat," *New York Times*, September 24, 1979, p. C-3.

pensate for the discrimination, and the employer may be enjoined from further violations of the Act.

2. Title VII of the Civil Rights Act of 1964 established a general prohibition against discrimination by sex (as well as race, religion, and national origin) in employment practices. The practices covered by this Title include hiring and firing, pay, classification of employees, and conditions of employment. However, employers were allowed to discriminate in hiring if sex was a "bona fide occupational qualification" for a particular job. Remedies for discrimination under Title VII generally are similar to those under the Equal Pay Act. Amendments in 1972 and 1978 expanded the coverage of this law and strengthened its prohibition of sex discrimination.

3. Executive Order 11375, issued by President Johnson in 1967, required guarantees against sex discrimination by employers contracting with the federal government. The Order amended an earlier Executive Order (11246) that prohibited racial discrimination by federal contractors. An employer that is found to discriminate can have current contracts with the federal government cancelled and can be declared ineligible for further federal contracts.

4. Title IX of the Education Amendments of 1972 is the major source of legal protection against sex discrimination in education, applicable to both students and school employees. With some exceptions, Title IX requires that "No person in the United States shall, on the basis of sex, be excluded from participation in, be denied the benefits of, or be subjected to discrimination under any education program or activity receiving Federal financial assistance..." Nearly all institutions of higher education and public elementary and secondary schools do receive such assistance. A violation of this requirement can be punished with a termination of federal aid.

These laws transform the legal status of women in organizations, and their potential impact is enormous. By their language, they seem destined to bring about essentially equal treatment for women as students and employees. Yet there are many forces that might limit the actual impact of these laws. In the next section I will explore the effect of these limiting forces.

II

People concerned with the problem of sex discrimination had reason to celebrate when laws such as Title VII were adopted. These laws created a national policy against certain forms of discrimination and established penalties for discriminatory behavior. Yet there also was good reason to be restrained in the celebration, for the history of laws which were intended to eliminate certain kinds of behavior indicated that such laws were not guaranteed success.

The most obvious example is the criminal laws. Although acts such as burglary and assault are punishable by imprisonment, they occur with depressing frequency. Even the threat of very severe penalties for the most serious crimes has not caused these crimes to disappear.

A closer parallel to the sex discrimination laws is the set of laws intended to provide full civil rights for black citizens. The array of constitutional provisions, statutes, and court decisions that prohibit racial discrimination have had only limited success. The Supreme Court's ruling in 1954 against separate schools for blacks and whites was largely unenforced in the Deep South for more than a decade. The Fifteenth Amendment's guarantee of voting rights for black citizens required a full century to become effective. Discrimination in employment and housing continues despite statutory prohibitions.

In the relatively few years that they have operated, the laws against sex discrimination also have proved to be less than fully effective. Discrimination in schools and in businesses continues to occur as much more than an isolated phenomenon. The apparent weaknesses of Title VII, Title IX, and the other laws in this field provide additional evidence of the law's limits as a mechanism to change people's behavior.

The reasons for these limits in the law's capacity are complex. But certainly the concept of deterrence is central to an understanding of the law's weaknesses as well as its strengths. Beyond whatever symbolic force it has, the law can cause people to change their behavior only by giving them incentives to change. More specifically, a law that prohibits people from doing something will be successful to the extent that it raises the costs that they expect to pay for doing it. The partial failures of criminal laws and civil rights laws result chiefly from their inability to punish prohibited behavior with sufficient certainty and severity.

Why is the deterrent impact of the laws against sex discrimination so imperfect? Many forces could be cited as part of the problem, but two merit emphasis: weaknesses in the administrative implementation of these laws, and the reluctance of some women to seek their rights under the laws.

The importance of administrative agencies as implementors of the law has become increasingly clear. Laws are not self-executing; they have to be put into effect in the administrative process. Moreover, the process of putting laws into effect is inherently imperfect and often fundamentally flawed. As a result, failures to achieve the goals of public policies often follow from implementation problems.

Certainly administrative agencies play central roles in implementing the laws against sex discrimination. Enforcement responsibilities have been given to several federal agencies. Title VII is carried out by the Equal Employment Opportunities Commission (EEOC). Since 1979 the EEOC also has had responsibility for enforcement of the Equal Pay Act; prior to that time the Act was handled by the Department of Labor. The Labor Department remains responsible for Executive Order 11375, through its Office of Federal Contract Compliance Programs; until 1978 it shared that task with the agencies that made contracts which were subject to the Order. The Office for Civil Rights of the Department of Education carries out Title IX, a job that it inherited from the Department of Health, Education and Welfare (HEW) upon creation of the new department.

The responsibilities of the various administrative agencies take several forms. They must write detailed regulations that give greater specificity to the general language of the statutes and executive order. Complaints of violations of the law generally go first to the appropriate agency for evaluation. If a complaint is found to have merit, the agency—depending upon the law—may initiate action in court to enforce the law or may act to enforce sanctions itself. Agencies also have some power and some legal obligation to monitor compliance with the laws even in the absence of complaints.

Most evaluations of the performance of administrative agencies in this field have been primarily negative. Critics have pointed to problems in each of the areas of administrative responsibility. Perhaps the most visible problem has been the great delay by some agencies in issuing regulations, which has slowed enforcement efforts. For instance, HEW did not issue final guidelines on sex discrimination in school athletics until December 1979, more than seven years after the adoption of Title IX. The problem of delay has been accompanied by other problems that are less visible, such as inadequate processing of discrimination complaints.

This is not to say that administrative handling of the sex discrimination laws has been uniformly bad. Certainly there are examples of vigorous and effective enforcement of these laws—and some critics have complained that particular laws are enforced too vigorously. But problems of implementation clearly have weakened the effects of the laws.

These problems derive from several causes, none of which is unique to this area of policy. One cause is the limited resources provided by Congress for some enforcement responsibilities, reflecting a common tendency in civil rights to give agencies sweeping mandates and little money to fulfill those mandates. The backlog of complaints that built up in the EEOC shortly after its creation was largely a product of the limited staff that was authorized for the agency. But resources have not been inadequate in all instances, and lack of money can explain only some enforcement problems.

Another cause of problems is the inefficiencies and inertia that seem to be endemic to bureaucratic organizations. HEW enforcement of Title IX, for instance, suffered from such familiar traits as poor coordination between national and regional offices and a fear of making definitive rulings that might produce criticism. Executive Order 11375 was originally to be enforced jointly by the Department of Labor and the contracting

agencies, and the agencies involved never coordinated enforcement efforts very well.
One major source of problems is a lack of will. In several instances, responsibilities for the enforcement of sex discrimination laws were given to agencies that had only a limited commitment to these laws. In the EEOC, enforcement of Title VII against sex discrimination initially suffered because some agency officials gave priority to race. In the case of Executive Order 11375, the problem was more fundamental. Federal agencies that allocate money to businesses and schools were told in effect to attack discrimination in these institutions. But to follow that course would have complicated the process of getting contract work done and would have interfered with working relationships between agency personnel and contractors. It appears that this was one major reason for the weakness of enforcement efforts by the contracting agencies.

By the late 1970s administrative problems seemed to have declined somewhat. Enforcement responsibilities were restructured, long-awaited regulations were issued, and some agencies showed increased commitment to their jobs. One reason for this improvement was the work of the women's movement in pressing for effective administrative agency. Another was the relatively favorable attitude of the Carter administration toward these laws. But administrative problems did not disappear. Moreover, the Reagan administration is less sympathetic to the laws against sex discrimination than its predecessors, and problems of limited resources and lack of will are likely to increase.[8]

Administrative problems reduce the law's deterrent effect by making it less likely that violations will be detected and punished. Because enforcement of the laws against sex discrimination have been quite imperfect, their potential effect on the behavior of company and university officials is limited. At the extreme, the virtual non-enforcement of the Executive Order for several years gave employers much less reason to

[8]In the first eighteen months of the Reagan administration there were several indications of a lessened commitment to legal attacks on sex discrimination, including appointments of officials to some enforcement agencies and proposed new regulations for Executive Orders 11246 and 11375.

pay attention to it.

A second force that has weakened the impact of these laws is the reluctance of some women to bring complaints under them. Like administrative weaknesses, this reluctance is not unique to this area of policy. Americans often are viewed as a litigious people, eager to take legal action when the opportunity arises. There is some truth to this image. But the vast majority of grievances that could be taken to court are not; in most instances, people live with their grievances or work them out informally. There are strong incentives to do so: the costs of legal action, the existence of simpler methods to resolve disputes, the uncertainty of outcomes in court, the adverse effect of legal action on people's relationships.

Each of these incentives is relevant to the use of laws against discrimination within organizations. The effect of legal action on relationships is worth special consideration. When a woman makes a formal complaint under the law, under most circumstances her bringing of the complaint becomes known to the people whom she has accused of discrimination — people who stand above her and have power over her in the organization. It is likely that her relationships with those people will become adversarial and unpleasant. Indeed, her position in the whole complex of relationships within the organization may become tenuous.

Some anti-discrimination laws prohibit retaliation against people who file complaints. But people in organizations often are so dependent upon discretionary judgments by their superiors that formal protections from retaliation may mean little. Certainly a middle-level business executive or a graduate student is highly vulnerable to subtle "punishment" for taking legal action. Some categories of people may be less vulnerable, including those who are protected by labor union membership or civil service status and those whose commitment to the organization is limited. But the woman who wants to stay in the organization and to move up, when the path up is highly unstructured, often has good reason to be concerned with the consequences of filing a complaint.

What if the complaint ultimately is successful, resulting in a favorable legal ruling or a settlement between the parties? The complainant's problems may not end at that point. The organization may balk at providing the relief that has been ordered or agreed upon. Even if it complies, however, the resentment and tension that resulted from the filing of a complaint are likely to continue. A study of employees who were reinstated to their jobs by the National Labor Relations Board found that relatively few actually returned to those jobs and remained for as long as two years; the major reason was the prospect or fact of retaliatory treatment by employers.[9] Similarly, women who win legal victories involving sex discrimination often suffer negative consequences within their organizations after the victories. As two social scientists have said about discrimination grievances generally, "victory may turn into defeat."[10]

These problems often produce unhappy outcomes for women who file complaints of sex discrimination. Perhaps more important, they discourage complaints by other women who observe or anticipate such outcomes. Ironically, it is the women who are most likely to suffer from discrimination, the ones who are most subject to discretionary decisions by people above them, that have the most to fear if they file complaints. The ultimate effect of discouraging complaints, of course, is to weaken the deterrent elements of the law by reducing the likelihood that sex discrimination will be challenged.[11]

III

Clearly, the laws which prohibit sex discrimination suffer from serious weaknesses in their operation. But this does not mean that these laws lack effect altogether. Again, the criminal statutes provide a useful analogy. The problems involved

[9]Les Aspin, "Reinstatement Isn't Enough," *American Federationist*, 78 (September, 1971), 19-21.

[10]Richard E. Miller and Austin Sarat, "Grievances, Claims, and Disputes: Assessing the Adversary Culture," *Law and Society Review*, 15 (1981-82), 541. There is a vivid summary of the problems that result from bringing a sex discrimination suit, even if the plaintiff is successful, in Jane O'Reilly, *The Girl I Left Behind* (New York: Macmillan, 1980), p. 136.

[11]One study found that people who felt that they had suffered from some form of discrimination were less likely to take legal action, or any other kind of action, than people with other types of grievances related to the law. Miller and Sarat, "Grievances, Claims, and Disputes," 536-546.

in carrying out these statutes, especially the difficulty of apprehending suspects, are tremendous. Because of these problems, the criminal laws cannot deter crime with anything like total effectiveness. Yet the criminal laws do work well enough to have *some* deterrent effect; certainly more crimes would be committed if there were no possible penalties attached to them.

In the same way, the laws against sex discrimination have some impact on discrimination. Despite all their imperfections, laws such as Title VII operate with a degree of effectiveness. As a result, they affect the treatment of women by company and university officials.

The impact of the sex discrimination laws arises first of all from the frequency with which complaints are made under these laws. In one year, for instance, the EEOC received more than 30,000 complaints of sex discrimination under Title VII.[12] Such a figure may be surprising in light of the risks that frequently are involved in filing complaints; it would seem to reflect both the frequency with which women feel that they have been subjected to discrimination and the fact that there are many women for whom the risks of using the law are minimal or who choose to ignore them.[13] In any case, large numbers of complaints are brought.

The bringing of a complaint in itself exacts costs from an organization. Officials need to take time and expend resources to respond to the complaint. For a small concern, even a few complaints may be quite burdensome. Even for a large corporation or university, a steady stream of complaints creates a real drain on organizational resources. As a result, officials have some incentive to change their operations in order to minimize the likelihood that complaints will be brought.

---

[12]U.S. Equal Employment Opportunity Commission, *Beginning the Second Decade: Eleventh Annual Report — Fiscal Year 1976,* p. 15.

[13]Some women may be able to join a group bringing a joint complaint or obtain administrative action without making an official complaint that exposes them to risks. Others may feel that they have nothing left to lose by bringing a complaint because their position in the organization has become untenable. Some complaints of discrimination are brought by people who feel that doing so actually will strengthen their position strategically even if the action ultimately is unsuccessful.

When a complaint is brought, of course, it may result in some penalties against the organization. Through formal decision or settlement women who have brought complaints may receive money awards, an organization may be required to change its practices, or it may suffer the loss of federal money.

From the perspective of people concerned with discrimination, the imposition of these penalties may seem all too rare. Indeed, the more severe the penalty under the law, the less that it seems to be used. The termination of federal funds and contracts under Title IX and Executive Order 11375, for instance, has been quite uncommon.

But employers and school officials necessarily take a different perspective. Even if major sanctions are unlikely to result from a particular complaint or administrative investigation, the mere possibility of such sanctions may be unsettling. A good example is a university that the Department of Labor investigates on the basis of sex discrimination complaints under Executive Order 11375. Past history indicates that such a university is fairly safe from the possibility that federal money will be cut off. But the results of a cutoff would be so disastrous that its possibility must be taken seriously.

Moreover, major sanctions for sex discrimination are not unknown. Even individual complaints may win large amounts of money. More important are the broader victories won as a result of class action suits or administrative initiatives. A few companies, for instance, have had millions of dollars of federal contract money cut off under Executive Orders 11246 and 11375. Class actions and consolidated administrative actions under Title VII also have resulted in major victories requiring the payment of large sums in damages and the establishment of general affirmative action plans to restructure employment.

The most significant of all these victories was the consent decree involving American Telephone and Telegraph Company, the nation's largest private employer of women.[14] EEOC, in conjunction with other federal agencies, responded to com-

[14]See Phyllis A. Wallace, ed., *Equal Employment Opportunity and the AT&T Case* (Cambridge: MIT Press, 1976); and Herbert R. Northrup and John A. Larson, *The Impact of the AT&T—EEO Consent Decree* (Philadelphia: Wharton School, University of Pennsylvania, 1979).

plaints of race and sex discrimination by seeking a massive remedy from AT&T. In 1973 a consent decree with the company was signed. The decree required the payment of tens of millions of dollars in compensation to women and members of racial minority groups. It also required a restructuring of employment patterns, with women recruited into previously male-dominated jobs and men into female-labelled jobs. The impact of the decree on AT&T as an employer was overwhelming.

The existence of such outcomes for discrimination complaints reinforces the perception by organization officials that they must act to reduce their vulnerability under the laws. This perception does not depend on an admission that the organization actually has engaged in discrimination. Officials may believe that complaints of discrimination generally are unfounded and malicious. They may perceive the administrative agencies that enforce the laws against discrimination as holding a bias against the organizations that they investigate. Even so, they may well feel a need to change their practices in order to insulate themselves from legal sanctions for discrimination.

One visible effect of this feeling is the proliferation of publications and seminars to train officials in the laws against discrimination and the requirements to avoid liability under them. Efforts to ensure equal opportunity have become a common subject of annual reports and other company literature. Perhaps most notable is the creation of offices for affirmative action in many large organizations.

All this activity does not indicate directly how much the incidence of discrimination has been reduced by the law. One way to examine this issue is in terms of women's general status as employees and students. If the law has brought about a serious decline in discrimination, then women's status should have improved as a result.

Indeed, women in work organizations and in schools have gained in some important respects — though not in all respects — since the laws against sex discrimination were adopted.[15] For instance, the numbers of women in some tra-

[15]One very important respect in which women have not gained is in the disparity between the median income of full-time working women and full-time working men. U.S. Department of Labor, *The Earnings Gap Between Women and Men* (Washington: Government Printing Office, 1979).

ditionally male occupations and in school athletic activities have grown dramatically. Clearly, much has changed in the last two decades.

It is difficult to ascertain the importance of the laws in bringing about these gains, because other forces also have played a part. The dramatic growth in female law school enrollment, for instance, probably reflects the impact of the law on school admissions and advising practices, but other factors such as changes in women's aspirations may be much more important. Efforts to separate out the impact of the law from other factors affecting women's employment status have produced conflicting results,[16] and the task would be no easier in education.

At the same time, some important effects of the law are fairly easy to identify. A good many women have been direct beneficiaries of legal victories such as the AT&T consent decree. In school athletics Title IX has been seen as the major impetus for expansion of women's programs, even with little effective enforcement of the law.[17] On the basis of these kinds of evidence, it seems clear that the law has made a real difference to women as students and employees.

Still, any tentative conclusions about the impact of federal laws must be mixed. The law has been one important force helping to bring about a reduction in discrimination against women and thus an improvement in their status. But it clearly has not eliminated discrimination altogether; sex discrimination remains a widespread organizational phenomenon, particularly in its subtler forms. Nor has it been responsible for all the gains that women have achieved in the past two decades; it is likely that other forces collectively have been far too powerful.

---

[16]Andrea H. Beller, "The Impact of Equal Employment Opportunity Laws on the Male-Female Earnings Differential," in Cynthia Lloyd, Emily S. Andrews, and Curtis L. Gilroy, eds., Women in the Labor Market (New York: Columbia University Press, 1979), pp. 304-330; Paul Burstein, "Equal Employment Opportunity Legislation and the Income of Women and Nonwhites," American Sociological Review, 44 (June 1979), 367-391.

[17]Women's basketball coaches in one informal survey agreed that Title IX was the primary impetus for improvement in the quality of their programs. Tim Warren, "New Players Bring Changes to Game," Washington Post, Nov. 24, 1981, p. C2.

IV

What does all this mean for the woman in a business or academic organization? First of all, she may be able to provide her own evidence as to the limits of the law. A woman who is subjected to discriminatory treatment even though the law outlaws discrimination knows that legal prohibitions in themselves do not cause problems to vanish.

Yet a woman in such an organization may be benefiting from the effects that the law does have. The woman who holds a position with American Telephone and Telegraph that effectively was limited to men a decade ago is a direct beneficiary of the consent decree between the company and EEOC. Even in companies and universitites that have not been subjected to legal sanctions, opportunities have opened and conditions improved for women as a result of the law.

It is not just the existence of laws against sex discrimination that makes a difference; it also is the ways in which they are interpreted and implemented. If the Reagan administration reduces the commitment of the federal government to enforcement of the laws against sex discrimination, few women may feel a direct and identifiable impact. But that reduced commitment might signal business and school officials that discrimination is less likely to result in legal penalties, and the treatment of women in some organizations could change in subtle but significant ways. Similarly, Supreme Court decisions that interpret provisions of Title VII seem remote from the everyday lives of women in organizations, but such decisions ultimately may affect the situations of a great many women.

At the beginning of this chapter I raised some general questions about the impact of the law on women in organizations. My answers have been tentative and mixed. Those answers are appropriate, I think because our knowledge about the law's effect is imperfect and because what we do know is mixed.

I have given some emphasis to the limits of the law as a force against discrimination, because those limits often are overlooked. But it also is important to keep in mind the significance of what has happened to the law in the past two decades. For most of our history the law accepted and even encouraged discrimination against women. Now we have laws that explicitly prohibit discrimination. Whatever effect these laws have, they have put government in the position of proclaiming support for equality rather than for inequality. That in itself is a revolutionary change.

Effective Interpersonal Communication for Women of the Corporation:

Think Like a Man, Talk Like a Lady...

Mary Ann Fitzpatrick

Introduction

During the past few years, a number of books and articles have been written for women about different aspects of communication in the organization. "How to" manuals have become best-sellers and books on new approaches to male and female roles in organizations have become household items. Most of these books propose a set of easy to follow rules and injunctions on how to be a better communicator. The authors assume that these rules can be followed with the same results by all individuals, regardless of age, sex or race. This work is best considered as communication science fiction rather than communication science. In communication science, authors take great care in specifying the conditions under which an individual can use certain types of communication behaviors. These authors know that rules have to be modified to fit different communication situations.

Communication science is usually unavailable to the general public. Scientific findings lie buried in sophisticated research reports, complicated theories, and a morass of academic rhetoric. Unlike communication science fiction which offers panaceas, communication science specifies that there are no magic formulas to make an individual a better communicator. The odds favoring success can, however, be greatly improved with skill and hard work.

73

In this paper, we will translate some of the work in communication science on effective communication in the organization. Effective communication has been discussed by communication scientists who study sex differences in communication and those who study communication competence. We will consider each of these topics as pursued by communication scientists. Based on their work, we will suggest what works when for women in the organization.

Sex Differences in Communication

Imagine this scene. You are walking down the street and you see, a short distance away, a new young mother of your acquaintance pushing a baby carriage. You are a little concerned as she comes closer, for you cannot remember whether the newborn is a boy or a girl. Hoping to catch a glimpse of pink or blue, your confidence fades as you finally meet. The baby is wearing yellow. Now you must ask, "Is it a boy or a girl?"

Have you ever wondered why you had to know the sex of the child before you could begin a conversation with its mother? The answer is that you change your communication behavior depending on whether the child is male or female. Sex is not only a biological attribute of an individual but a social and emotional one as well. We are uncomfortable in not knowing the sex of an individual, no matter how young, for we do not know how to respond to them socially or emotionally without that vital piece of information.

As society changes, the social and emotional meaning of what it is to be a male or a female changes also. The social changes that our society has undergone in the past twenty years have renewed interest in understanding male and female differences. Much has been written about how men and women differ in their communication behaviors.

Those communication scientists who study sex differences in interpersonal behavior are, however, limited by the statistical techniques they use. Most of the statistical models that are used focus on testing and finding *differences* between people and ignore similarities. An example of this phenomenon is a study that I completed over four years ago. The study examined male and female perceptions of their own communication behavior as well as the behavior of one's best-same and opposite sex friend. Included in the interpersonal behavior examined were at least ten dimensions of behavior ranging from control to nurturance. Of the ten behaviors, males and females were significantly different on only *two*. The entire discussion section of the paper focused on the two differences uncovered between males and females.

Although there is a need for the kind of communication research that documents the differences between the interpersonal behaviors of males and females, the question of whether men are really more controlling or aggressive than women or whether women are really more expressive or emotional than men does not suggest how individuals can be more effective communicators. This cataloguing of sex differences leaves unanswered the question of what works when for women in the organization.

Communication Competence

In addition to sex differences in communication, communication scientists study what makes a competent communicator. A competent communicator is one who can accurately perceive his/her environment and can create and understand messages in light of these perceptions. The competent communicator can successfully accomplish his/her goals in a situation without embarrassing others or putting them down.

What does this mean? Good communicators are perceptive about other people and about the situations in which they find themselves. Not only are they sensitive to others but good communicators also have a variety of communication skills that allow them to accomplish their goals.

We have three separate and sometimes competing goals each time we communicate. The first is a task goal — get the job done. The job may be anything from hiring the right applicant, to explaining your position to others, to describing a new data system. The second goal is a relational goal — do not do unnecessary damage to the relationship between you and others by this message. Every time you communicate with others in the organization, you are making statements about the relationship you have to them. Do you call your boss: Sir, Joe,

Mr. Smith, or Smithie? Each of these ways of addressing him comments on the relationship that you have with him. The final goal in a communication situation is the identity management goal—make your communication project the image that you want. Every time you communicate with others in the organization, you are making statements about the kind of person you are. While our verbal behavior is more important when the goals of our interaction are task ones, nonverbal behaviors are especially crucial for relational and impression-management goals.

In a number of communication situations, each of these three goals—task, relational and identity management—can be accomplished by complementary verbal and nonverbal behavior. At times, however, the goals may be competing with one another. In other words, the communication behaviors used to accomplish a task may hinder a relational goal or even an impression-management goal. We will return to this point in a later section.

Once a communicator has a particular goal, he or she must choose from a variety of verbal and nonverbal behaviors the appropriate behaviors to reach the goal. One of three models of behavior is suggested for male and female communicators. The first is the masculine model. This model says that women in organizations should communicate like men. Women should focus on task goals and impression management goals to the exclusion of relational goals. The second is the feminist model. This model argues that men in organizations should communicate like women. Men should place greater emphasis on relational goals to the exclusion of task goals. The third is the androgynous model. This model suggests that men and women should blend their communication styles. Each should adopt communication behaviors of the other. Task and relational goals are predominant.

The androgyny model has been hailed as the answer to the business person's prayer. Be androgynous (capable of using male and female communication behaviors) because androgyny represents "the upper range of a general social competency dimension." In the seventies, androgyny became synonymous with the notion of the competent communicator. Androgynous people were capable of being assertive and dominant (task behaviors) and warm and nurturant (relational behaviors) in their interactions with others in the organization.

More recently, however, communication scientists found that androgyny has different outcomes for males and females. The adoption of masculine task behaviors enhances a female's adaptability while the adoption of feminine, relational behaviors proves problematic for males. Women who communicated like men did better in a variety of social situations. The healthiest and best-liked individuals, male or female, were assertive, decisive, and intellectual, rather than nurturant, responsive, and emotional.

Women are both perceived as better communicators and see themselves as better communicators when they adopt masculine communication patterns. This does not suggest that women in organizations need to cut their hair, deepen their voices and wear pants. What the research does show is that the communication characteristics that define masculinity are those associated with competence while those which define femininity are those associated with warmth and expressiveness. The characteristics that no one finds desirable are those defined as feminine characteristics.

The masculine model predicts communication success for both men and women of the organization better than the feminist or androgynous models. Women need to focus on task and impression-management goals in their interaction. These communication goals can be achieved using a variety of strategies. The legitimacy of some tactics for achieving task and impression-management goals may differ for males and females. An example may clarify this point.

Imagine you are in charge of a decision-making group in your organization. Your task is to lead the group to the successful completion of a project. Linguists suggest that individuals who use tag questions ("That's an interesting idea, isn't it?") or disclaimers ("I could be mistaken, but..."; "This may sound strange but...") are perceived as incompetent. Recent research in decision-making groups clearly shows that in using these expressions as they are working on a task, women are perceived as incompetent but men are perceived as polite.

While tag questions and disclaimers make men appear more socially competent, they merely make women appear uncertain. The example shows that while the overall communication strategies that men and women adopt in the communication may be the same, the tactics used by women must differ from those used successfully by men. The answer to what works when for women in the organization differs significantly from what works when for men.

Principles of Effective Communication

Have you ever had this experience? After a long and tiring day at the office, you get into your car to drive home. Forty minutes later, you pull into the driveway but *you do not remember anything about the trip.* How could this happen?

Since you have taken the route home many times, you drove home automatically, without thinking. You have a script for driving home. Scripts are sequences of events expected by an individual involving him/her or either a participant or the observer. If there is no deviation in the typical sequence, e.g. no roadblocks, detours or accidents, you are not even very aware that you are driving.

Much of our interpersonal communication is like that drive home. We have developed scripts that tell us what to say and in what order or how to respond and in what way. And we manage to engage in these scripts without paying much attention to what we are saying. Male and female scripts, especially concerning appropriate communication behavior in an organization, are very different. Males have highly routinized scripts for appropriate communication behaviors in an organization. They can use these scripts automatically, without devoting much thought or energy to them. Females, on the other hand, have no such ready-made organizational scripts. Indeed, the automatic responses they do have are very different from males. The female script in this culture specifies the inhibition of aggression and the open display of sexual urges, passivity with men although not with women, nurturance, and the cultivation of personal attractiveness. In communication, this is translated into emotional responsiveness, social poise, and a friendly posture with others. In communication, the masculine script is depicted by aggressiveness, independence in problem-solving, control of repressive urges, and suppression of strong negative emotions, especially anxiety.

The feminine script suggests giving rewarding responses and expects to receive rewarding responses. It places more emphasis on relational goals in interaction. The masculine script focuses on task and identity management goals first.

Without being aware of it, women in organizations are constantly set on a path of what we call in communication theory, transactional disqualification. Graphically stated, you are damned if you do and damned if you don't. One can be feminine thus incompetent or one can be competent thus masculine. Automatic scripted responses are not task-effective for women in the organization.

Since her automatic responses will generally be incorrect in the organizational environment, the first principles of effective communication for women in an organization is to analyze the situation carefully. There are five dimensions of communication on which these situations may vary. Situations may be competitive or cooperative, dominant or equal, intense or superficial, task-oriented or non-task oriented and formal or informal. Before you can decide on appropriate conduct within an interaction, you have to define the various aspects of that interaction.

In attempting to define a particular situation, ask yourself these five questions. (1) Cooperative versus Competitive: Are there no attempts made to persuade others or many attempts made to persuade others? (2) Dominance versus Equality: Is one person talking more than another or does neither person talk more than another? (3) Intense versus Superficial: Are individuals deeply engrossed in what is happening or very emotional or are they relatively involved and unemotional? (4) Task versus Nontask: Are there very clear goals or not very clear goals in this interaction? (5) Formal versus Informal: Are the individuals very reserved and cautious or very frank and open in their interactions?

Once you have defined the particular communication situation, then you need to think about what people are symbolically exchanging with one another as they communicate. In a communication exchange, each tries to get the most from the exchange that he/she can. One principle guiding the calculation of how appropriate an interpersonal exchange has been is an evaluation of the resources that have been exchanged. As we communicate with others, we are capable of exchanging love, status, information, money, goods, and services. Indeed, these are communication currency. When we offer one of these resources in communication, we expect reciprocation in kind. If we give status to another, then we expect respect in return. If we do not receive the same resource, we expect the one most closely allied to it in the list. In an organization, if we respect our boss, we expect him then to give us information and money in return.

Our messages acquire meaning when they are placed into one of these six resource classes. The more similarly two people code specific communication behaviors into classes, the fewer communication problems they have. If each communicator sees a particular piece of behavior as a status message, they have achieved a degree of understanding. A classic example of the coding of different behaviors into classes is that of organizational perquisites. Every organization has goods, e.g., a centrally located office, special drapes and rugs, charge accounts, etc. that are given to certain individuals. These goods are actually status messages. Some members are aware of the actual meaning of the receipt of these goods while others are not.

Traditionally, women have been largely restricted to trade in the resources of love that depend on personal relationships while men control concrete resources like money, information and physical strength. With the predominance of exchanging effect and relational goal enhancement, women code behavior and the rules for appropriate exchange differently than men. Men strongly differentiate love from status and information while women confuse the boundaries between these three resources. A woman feels bad when criticized for an idea (mild denial of status) because she codes it more personally as a denial of love or affect.

Differences in defining situations and in coding messages into resource classes clearly have profound impact on communication behavior between the sexes and on perceptions of the other's competence. If each sex has disparate presumptions about what constitutes appropriate behavior in context and if each is basing his/her assessment of the other's resource exchange preferences on his/her own, each is more likely to feel that the other's interpersonal communication behavior is ineffective. One manager expressed well the frustration he felt in dealing with women in his organization. "It's like they are from a different culture. It is hard to talk to them (women). I never know how they are going to react."

Since men and women place communication messages in different classes, it is easy to see why this manager feels as if women were from another culture. Most of the difficulty occurs with the information, status and love resources. These resources are more directly tied to the relationship between the communicators. Since males and females place different emphasis on relational goals, these resources are often miscoded. Women make fewer discriminations among love, status and information messages. Obviously, this leads to a number of communication difficulties.

Interaction Management

Both the definition of the situation and the placing of messages into one of the six resource classes are cognitively-mediated aspects of interaction. Once the appropriate cognitive choices have been made, women need to behave in a way that brings off a professionally rewarding communication performance. To do this, women need to manage their interaction.

Interaction management involves two interrelated sets of skills. The first is the ability to control an interaction without dominating it. This implies *mutual* control to insure that both participants achieve their goals. The second involves the ability to maintain a smooth and easy flow of interaction through the "procedural" aspects of structuring a conversation. Interaction management is the "smooth synchronization of speaking turns as evidenced by no attempts at simultaneous turns, no pauses in the conversation of three seconds or longer...and bilateral topic control" (Wiemann, 1977, pp. 201-202). There is a strong relationship between effective communication and interaction management. Total reciprocity of topic change and topic extension result in the highest ratings of competence and attraction. Conversations in which one person had substantially more or less than an equal share of turns for changing or extending topics were rated as incompetent.

Both men and women are incompetent when communicating with one another. Rather than mutual control, men do nearly all of the interrupting, are responsible for most lapses, and dominate floor time, while women allow this to occur. Although neither dominance nor submission are effective communication styles, a simple increase in domineering male interpersonal behaviors is not the solution. What will help women achieve their task and impression-management goals? Since the female script automatically tells women how to be emotionally responsive and nurturant, we will consider a few alternative ways for women to achieve control in a conversation.

To get the floor in a discussion, speakers raise their voices. Given their generally lower volume, higher voice pitch, and the likelihood of being socially sanctioned for using obvious control strategies, women should not raise their voices. To gain control of a situation, women can creatively use strategic questioning. The careful use of questions in a conversation controls when a topic is changed and when a topic is extended and discussed at greater length. Questions specify the range of appropriate responses that others may give and therefore structure and control the content of a conversation. Open-ended questions such as "How is the project going?" allow the respondent to say whatever he/she likes at whatever length he/she chooses. Closed questions, a form of question that greatly narrows the respondent's answer ("When can we expect the report of the data structures?"), allow the speaker to control the direction of the conversation.

To achieve their professional task and impression-management goals, women need to examine not what they say but how they say when they say. Verbal forms that imply tentativeness such as tag questions, qualifiers and disclaimers should be avoided.

Women also need to resist interruptions in conversations. Once a woman has the floor, she should resist giving it to another speaker until she has completed her points. At times, she may have to request the assistance of a colleague (another woman, a sympathetic male) to insure that her points are made. This same colleague might also be quietly enlisted to extend the topics that a woman initiates in a discussion. When we speak, our words may be accepted, rejected or ignored. An extensive body of research indicates that it is far better to be rejected or ignored.

Finally, women need to be careful that they are not undercutting what they say with their actions. When verbal and nonverbal messages are contradictory, individuals believe the nonverbal messages. To maintain control, women should adopt a slightly more relaxed posture, less frequent smiling (and smile only when there is something to smile about), nodding, head tilting and dropping of your eyes in response to another's gaze. Finally, women have to avoid using the intonation of a question (raising the voice at the end of a sentence rather than lowering it) when making a declarative statement.

Changing verbal behavior is easier than changing nonverbal behavior. One successful technique is videotaping yourself at meetings, in discussions, or giving presentations. Many corporations make such facilities available. Seeing how you communicate is a first step in deciding what behaviors need work. If such facilities are unavailable to you, seek feedback from a close colleague. Ask if you ever send inconsistent messages? Do you nod or smile at incorrect times?

Competent interaction is not achieved by the simple repetition of the same behavioral control patterns utilized by the other interactant. Indeed, to return in kind, interruption for interruption, long speech for long speech, severely mitigates against the "smooth and easy flow of interaction." That, after all, is what we are striving for.

Conclusion

There is an old adage that best sums up what I have tried to say to women of the organization: Think like a man, talk like a lady, and work like a dog. Think like a man. Define the communication situation like a man would and code messages as he would. Talk like a lady. Use alternative techniques to get the floor, to make your point and to assure yourself credit for your ideas. Work like a dog. Margaret Mead, a noted anthropologist, once remarked that although it was far more difficult for women to achieve success in the organizations of America than for men, women had to do the necessary work. Women must become more influential in modern organizations for they bring a needed and unique perspective.

We communicate with others either to understand them or to influence them. Influencing people and events is more important in organizations than is understanding them. Indeed, in organizational life, understanding others is only a means to an end. The end is influence.

Women have well-developed scripts for understanding others. Women need to create such scripts for influencing others. The work from communication science should help in the development of those scripts and the improvement of inter-personal communication in the organization.

Breakthrough: Making It Happen with Women's Networks

Sue DeWine

Every Monday at noon, 12 very powerful individuals meet in Chicago. Over lunch they exchange business tips and pass along mutually useful information for their respective firms. When job openings occur at their organizations, these individuals share this information with each other *first*. Included in this meeting are the following individuals: President of a direct marketing division for a major manufacturer, Medical Director for a pharmaceutical company, Executive Vice President for an investment agency, International Vice President of a food products firm, Vice President for a large retail chain, Vice President for a state utilities company, and corporate Vice President for a major publishing company. These individuals negotiate business deals among themselves that can have millions of dollars of impact for their organizations.

In Milwaukee, Wisconsin another group meets every third Thursday of the month with a very restrictive membership. A recruiting committee seeks only top ranking executives from corporations and the group allows one individual per 500 employees from any one type of business. They have developed a packet of materials to be distributed to other individuals wanting to form such a group.

In Columbus, Ohio a similar group meets once every two months for the purpose of making professional contacts as well as sharing career information on a variety of topics. This group meets without any restrictions on membership. Any individual may attend these meetings and pay per-meeting dues.

What these groups have in common is that they are all examples of women's networks. These women are doing
something men have always done very naturally-develop an
"Old Boys' Network." Men's networking occurs more often as
a by-product of membership in social clubs, civic organizations, and participation in athletic events. Women, on the other
hand, are establishing different methods for facilitating contacts. They have formalized this informal activity by establishing overt freestanding networks. It is a deliberate strategy to
link women with other women in an attempt to expand contacts, provide successful role models for each other, generate
solutions to problems, and disseminate information. The names
vary and include: "The Columbus Women's Network" in
Columbus, Ohio; "Tempo: An Organization for Executive,
Management and Professional Women" in Milwaukee,
Wisconsin; "Women's Lunch Group" in Boston; "Women in
Business" located in Los Angeles; "Women's Forum" in
Denver; "Forum for Executive Women" in Philadelphia; and
the "Executive Women's Club" in Pittsburgh. *Working Woman*
has published a list of hundreds of women's networks across
the country in a 1981 issue of the magazine. Although the
names vary, the intent of these professional networks is to put
women in contact with other women who may be able to help
them advance their careers. Perhaps you're wondering exactly
what women do when they are involved in the process of "networking"? What kinds of behaviors are expected?

What is "Networking"?

Professional networking is a process of *linking people to each
other as career resources;* and assisting, supporting and
helping others to find the resources they need. This is different
from "support groups" which are groups that meet to help one
another cope with some psychological or physiological problem (like Network of Battered Wives) or meet because they
share some common religious or political belief (like the National Organization for Women). Support groups serve other purposes .and advance individual's careers only indirectly. Professional career networks are established for the specific purpose of advancing women in their chosen career-helping

women cope with some of the professional issues discussed earlier in this book. The motivation for joining professional networks is to make contacts with other individuals who can help you develop your career path. The following examples illustrate how this might happen.

> The Personnel Director of a large industrial firm is planning to leave. Before she tells her boss about her resignation she tells a potential successor, who then starts lining up support for her application before the job is even posted.

> A woman is interviewing for a top-level job and needs to know what kind of salary she should expect at this level and with this particular firm. With the information she gets from other networkers she is able to negotiate successfully for one of the highest paid positions in the firm. Without access to the right information she might very well have settled for a much lower salary.

> A woman in business for herself calls on a fellow networker who is a loan officer in a local bank and learns first hand from a fellow colleague, what are the best types of loans currently available.

The topic of networking has exploded in the popular literature in the past three years. Articles on networking have appeared in major women's magazines or news journals throughout the country. Two authors who have written extensively about this phenomenon are Mary Scott Welch and Carol Kleiman.[1] Welch provides an excellent review of the concept of networking as a strategy for career development. She identifies networking as "The process of developing and using your contacts for information, advice, and moral support as you pursue your career."

Kleiman has divided the networks she has studied into six major categories: business, professional support, health/ sports, political/labor, and artistic. Some of these "networks" would be included under the category of support groups as defined for this article. Kleiman also notes that there are many informal networks that have and will continue to evolve as women increase their contacts and become more

[1]Welch, M.S. *Networking: The great new way for women to get ahead.* New York: Harcourt, Brace & Jovanovich, 1980. And, Kleiman, C., *Women's networks.* New York: Lippincott & Crowell, 1980.

aware of each other's needs. A professional network has been described by one networker in the following way: "Members are not allowed to talk about their kids, their husbands, or their emotional crises. We don't want people who are finding themselves or searching out new life styles. We are interested in people who can contribute to each other in the marketplace." This particular networker founded a women's network in Boston that meets monthly at the Harvard Club.

This chapter will examine these career orientated networks by identifying some of the motivations behind their development, positive and negative impacts of their activities for both the network member and her organization, and specific steps and techniques for establishing a network of your own. From a communication specialist's point of view this phenomenon has implications for the ways in which individuals communicate with one another within the organization as well as outside the organization in essentially working relationships.

Why Join a Professional Network?

Professional women have often had difficulty making use of informal and formal networks within, as well as external, to their organizations. As more women reach middle and top level management positions in organizations, they have found that *useful contacts are unavailable* to them and have begun to establish their own networks in response to their need for links with others who can help them professionally. The extent to which a network can do this varies. In a 1981 case study of one women's network by Casbolt and DeWine[2] women were asked what their goals and objectives were in joining the women's network. Most of the women in this midwestern professional network responded that their primary objective in participating in the network was to get career information and to make contacts with other women. The lowest ranked objective was to seek other women to fill job openings. Clearly this network has

[2]Casbolt, D. & DeWine, S. Inter Organizatinal Networks: Formal Communication Systems of Female Organizational Members. Paper presented at the International Communication Association, May 1981 in Mineapolis, Minnesota.

more women participants who need other's help than it has women who have positions to fill. Depending on the structure of the network itself, women may be joining together to collectively seek out resources or to assist each other professionally in a mutually satisfactory way.

I would *not* suggest that women should ignore access, however limited, to already established networks either in their own organization or professional affiliations. In attitude research some women have indicated that rather than plug into informal networks they felt they should back off, thinking they should form a women's network instead. If your main reason for networking with women is to avoid having to cope with entering existing networks, then networking may be a mistake. Such support groups are valuable in their own right, but they cannot replace working with individuals, male and female, in the system in which you are located. I *would* suggest that establishing a women's network more overtly will *assist you in advancing your career more quickly.*

Networks also *reduce some of the isolation* that women often feel on the job and increase their sense of participation and self confidence. As one woman put it, "Having my firm hire another woman for a position we have open would not really change my job in any way but would simply provide me with a professional in my immediate environment who might be able to identify more readily with my needs and concerns."

Overcoming isolation can be a reason for networking *within* the organization as well as networking *across* organizations. Another reason for networking across organizations rather than internally is the *difficulty women may have in finding other women in their own organization to establish contact with.* The Gallagher Reports indicate that of the 100 highest paid US marketing company or advertising agency executives *no* women were included. Forbes' 1979 annual survey of 803 chief executive officers of the largest US companies did not include one woman. A survey of 1,300 top fortune companies revealed that only 10 women held high ranking office or director positions. The University of Wisconsin at Milwaukee conducted a study titled, "Women in Top Jobs in Milwaukee" and concluded that there were none in Milwaukee! A severe shortage of women in top management who can serve as role models or mentors to women in lower management levels may deter the progress of those who depend on them for developmental support. With so few women in top level management positions it would seem a necessity that women network across organizational boundaries.

A most important reason why many women participate actively in networks is that a *majority of jobs come through personal contacts.* For example, Jane Keller knew a female colleague was applying for a position with the National Abortion Rights Action League and put her in touch with another woman who was conducting an extensive case study of the NARAL's publicity campaign. The job applicant was able to use the results of the recent research to suggest new publicity directions for NARAL as a part of her interviewing responses. It helped her demonstrate her ability to collect new ideas and put them to practical use. She got the job! And Jane Keller got a future contact who would be willing to give her information when she needed it.

The US Bureau of Labor indicates that at least 48% of job leads come from personal contacts and the higher up the executive ladder the more jobs are filled by word of mouth. Recently, I tried to obtain information about a high ranking position with an organization for a colleague who was interested in moving to the area in which I was living. Two days after I had tried calling individuals responsibile for the position and getting very little information, my husband came home from a Kiwanis meeting where the position had been described in detail for fellow Kiwanians who might know persons interested in applying for the position. If women do not establish networks of their own to counter limited access to such informal grapevines they will continue to be left out of top level management positions. We also know that women working full time earned on an average, 59 cents for every dollar earned by a man and the gap between female and male earnings has been widening, not decreasing. Welch reports the following startling statistics:

> We're 42 percent of the labor force, but we have nowhere near 42 percent of the good jobs. Eighty percent of us are still concentrated in lower-paying, lower-status jobs-in service industries, clerical fields, retail sales, manufacturing plants. Where

5,377 men were making $25,000 a year or more in 1977, the latest year for this particular breakdown of figures, only 2,000 women were in that income bracket. That year the average annual earnings of full-time women workers were $9,535, only 56% of men's average annual earnings of $16,929. That wage gap was greater still in sales, where women earn 45 cents of the men's dollar. Even in clerical work, "women's work," women earn less than men: female clericals earn 61 cents for every dollar earned by male clericals (In 1956, women in clerical occupations earned 72 percent of what their male counterparts were earning; in 1962, 69 percent; in 1976, 64 percent. They've come a long way-down).

We're 99 percent of all secretaries, hold fewer than 2 percent of the seats on the top 1,300 corporations' boards of directors. Sixteen percent of us are classified as "professional and technical workers" but whereas women professionals tend to be school teachers or nurses, men are lawyers, doctors, or college professors. As for managers and administrators, the category where we're supposed to be making such huge strides, we're only 6.3 percent of those. Managers and administrators are 93.7 percent male.

Men have learned to be competitive in such a way that the process taught them to compromise, cooperate, and collaborate. The same process teaches young girls how to win as *individuals* only, and to distrust other females. Women are now beginning to see the disadvantage that places them in. Networks provide very specific payoffs for women like: information, referrals, feedback, professional growth, and increased visibility. Along with the payoffs there can be some negative consequences that women must guard against.

Some Traps of Networking

One of the major objections raised concerning women's networks was alluded to earlier — men, *the very resource that women need to tap, are left out of most networks.* Is it useful for women to network with other women when the people who have the resources and the information they need to advance their careers may very well be men? And besides, aren't women then creating another system just like the one they are objecting to? These concerns are certainly valid and every

women's network needs to address them carefully in light of
the goals for that particular network. The fact is there are a
wide variety of types of networks that have been developed by
and for women but not necessarily restricted to women. A
female financial analyst at Equitable Life Assurance Society in
New York started an in-house network with the principle goals
of: opening informal channels for information exchange both
within and among Equitable's departments, enabling the organization to take full advantage of its human resources, and
helping members to form groups for support information or
business. At the request of a group of men the membership now
includes 10% men, many of whom "never had their own networks or if they did it was clear that they weren't fulfilling
career planning needs or that they were misused or under-
used." Although most women's networks that have been identified in national publications are restricted to women, there is
no reason that the concept that started as a focus for women
cannot be a focus for any group of individuals who feel that
they have limited access to informal networks currently in
operation in their particular setting. It is important that the
network participants constantly revaluate their particular
goals and objectives and structure the membership according-
ly. Limiting membership to only top level executives or managers, whether they are men or women, is another objection
raised by critics of women's networks.

Is it fair for women to limit their membership to only other
women who have achieved the same rank or higher level in
organizations thus leaving out clerical workers and others at
the lowest levels of the organization? Networks vary on this
issue. Some, like "tempo," mentioned in the beginning of this
article, restrict their membership to the highest ranking
women in major organizations. Their feeling is that in order for
a network to be useful to you, you must be making contact with
other women who will be doing your career the most good.
Otherwise, women in top level positions will find that they end
up giving free consulting advice on a continual basis if the network is made up of women from all levels of the organization.
On the other hand, if the network's primary goal is dissemination of information, like the "Columbus Women's Network,"
then anyone who can make use of the information should be

able to attend. The founders of this network feel that the nature of the topics discussed and the type of information disseminated will allow women to screen themselves out if the information is not as useful to them. There are those who would say, "If you aren't part of the solution then you may be part of the problem." If women aren't willing to help other women beneath them advance to higher positions in the organization then can these same women legitimately argue that the present system limits the amount of contact they have with informal channels of information? On the other hand, if networks are to be useful to you it would seem that you need to ensure that the contacts you will make will be with individuals in positions of more responsibility and authority than yourself or at least with an equal level of responsibility so that you can learn from them how to move through the organization. You need to determine for yourself what your specific objectives are in participating in a network and be sure that those objectives are being met. If they aren't then it is your responsibility and no one elses, to do something about it. One writer has suggested that women may want to network with other women at their own level or higher thus restricting network membership but additionally helping other women obtain professional advancement by occasionally having open meetings where the network members act as consultants free of charge to women in entry level positions.

The case study by Casbolt and DeWine raised the issue of appropriate use of women's networks. In that particular study the women who were most involved in the formal network were less involved in the act of networking *outside* the formal group. Women who had dropped out of the formal network reported making more professional contacts (80% compared to approximately 37% of the network participants who actively made professional contacts outside the formal network). One could raise the question that perhaps *the ones using the network the most are the individuals least able to be effective* at it and those who are effective at making contacts do so on their own without the aid of a formal network activity. However, the particular network studied was one that did not have restrictive membership. As a consequence, few top level executive women were members. Perhaps the women who were not members, or had dropped out of the network, were the very ones this group needed to seek out. Additionally, many women report using a women's network to help them initially see ways to advance their career and once they've gained the informa-tion they need, at least temporarily, they move out of that "external" system and move more solidly into an "internal" communication system within their own organization.

There is some evidence that networking does actually help advance careers. In a sample of 400 male and female workers in a national financial institution a number of variables were examined (age, race, meetings with supervisor, education, per-ceived importance of skills, formal system information, grape-vine information, and personal contacts) and women's use of personal contacts was the greatest predictor of promotion and higher salary.[3] It would seem that as women's skill of using and making professional contacts increase the potential for career advancement is likely to increase. However, for many, this proof is not substantial yet and the true value of women's net-working activities remains untested.

Two fears expressed by employers about networking activities are that they *may promote the sharing of confidential information or worse become a vehicle for unionization at-tempts.* While both of these are possible outcomes of any in-formal or formal communication system, giving away company secrets is not compatible with career development within the company. One of the things a new networker might very well learn from the network itself is what type of information is pub-lic and what type essentially stays within a division or unit. Just as the "Old Boys' Network" has developed ways of guiding colleagues in their careers without giving away confidential in-formation, the "new girls' networks" are learning the same technique. For example, when Barb James, a customer relations officer for a retail department store, was offered pro-motions in two of the store's divisions — corporate development and marketing — she was unsure of which to accept. She called a female colleague in the business office whom she had met at

[3]Stewart, L. Upward Communication and Other Factors Influencing the Promotability of Males and Females within an Organization. Paper presented at the International Communication Association, May 1981 in Minneapolis, Minnesota.

a career development seminar and asked for advice. Over lunch the two women discussed the offers. James' co-networker had access, because of her position, to information about future directions for the company and she knew, although James did not, that the corporate development division had been identified by top management as an area for expansion in the coming year. She encouraged James to take the offer from corporate development indicating that she thought more opportunities would be available later but *without* disclosing any confidential information. Six months later when James' department was looking for a new financial analyst she told her colleague, who had been so helpful to her, about the opening. James' colleague, through this early access to information, applied for and got the job.

As for networks being a vehicle for unionization, that is a possibility where the goal of the network activity is to discuss issues like inadequate benefits or poor working conditions. Where the goal is career development, the possibility that an internal network will result in some union activity is quite remote. It is the responsibility of individuals interested in the network to determine appropriate goals and objectives. If the internal networks want the support of management it will be crucial that participants carefully outline for their respective organizations the focus on career and professional advancement.

Finally, regardless of the values of networking, there are *individuals who will abuse the practice* which makes those with the most to contribute to a network wary of involvement with it. If an individual joins in networking activities expecting to broker" her skills or give them to the "highest bidder" this can sabotage the system. If a woman attempting to advance her career expects that other women who have "made it" *owe* her their assistance, this can sabotage the system. And if network members whose careers are just beginning feel that there is nothing they can offer that would be useful to anyone else, this too can sabotage the system. Susan Peck's experience is an example of this type of abuse. Susan is a corporate executive and one of the founders of a Chicago network. Soon after starting the network she received a phone call from a woman she had never met who said, "I belong to your network and I'd like for you to set up some interviews for me at your firm. I want to move into a position of more authority—more power." Without any other contact this caller is taking advantage of Peck's demonstrated concern to help women advance their careers. Another woman new to networking, told a prominent speaker at her networking meeting that she had given her name as a job reference. "I figured you wouldn't mind since you're so supportive of women."

Networking must be two sided with mutual respect for all parties. The best way to network is to offer some skill or information to someone first before requesting their help. The secret to networking is to always be alert to ways in which you may be able to help someone else's career. It may be as simple as letting another female employee in your organization know that this week would be a good time to ask for a raise since you happen to know that budget reports just came out positively, or letting a female colleague know about a job opening that has not been posted yet. People who get high ranking jobs usually find out about them long before they are publicly advertised. You can find ways to be helpful to others both below and above you in the organizational hierarchy. If someday you need to draw on the relationship you developed because of your assistance, you already have "credit" with this colleague. However, keep in mind that networking is a system of mutual support, not payoffs.

So You Want to Start a Network?

You're convinced that "networking" would be useful to you and your career but you're wondering how you should go about starting a network of your own. Whether you end up with a formal network with recognized members or you simply put into practice the principles of networking to establish your own private network, you should begin by building up a wide range of relationships. In essence, you *make every contact count*. Start by making a list of everyone you know, regardless of age, locale, position or degree of friendship. Unless you have been living in a very remote part of the world, your list should be well over 100 people. By each person's name begin to think of ways in which they might be helpful to you and your career. Do they *work in a field related* in any way *to your own career* interests? Or do they *work for an organization* that you might one day be interested in? Do they have *contacts* that you would like to make your own? Do they have *skills* you would like to learn? Do they have *knowledge or information* that would be helpful? Or perhaps they have a *style of relating to people* that you would like to study. Perhaps some of the names on your list are good friends who *provide* the *emotional support* anyone needs to take career as well as personal risks.

Multiply the number of contacts you have listed by 10 and you begin to see the potential of a network of just 10 other women! If you link with other women you automatically expand your contacts far beyond the number you could establish on your own. Once you have established trust with fellow networkers and you begin to understand the professional needs of one another the potential for professional contacts is only limited by your own imagination.

After identifying potential contacts your next step is to *track leads.* Keep some type of filing system on the people you meet who could be of some potential career help. Small note cards in a file might be convenient. Be sure to list the following: full name and title along with preferred nickname or shortened version of name, where and when you met the person, information exchanged, any promises you made to follow up, and ways in which you might be able to help them (i.e. type of job or contact they want to make) as well as ways in which they might be able to help you at some future date. When calling this person in the future refer to this card so that you can identify where you met them and ask specific questions that they may be able to answer.

Once you have begun making professional contacts more consciously begin to plan how to *incorporate them into your daily routine.* Examine your appointment book—how many dates with persons of value to your career have you made in the last month? If you have an appointment book that carefully keeps track of who and where you meet with professional associates you are at least making the first step. Examine previous entries and count up the number of times *you have initiated contact* with someone you thought might be helpful in advancing your career. You should average two luncheon meetings a week that you have initiated for the purpose of some career development step. One networker carries a small notebook with her that includes information on professional projects that she is currently working on so that any new piece of information or person she meets that could help her with that project gets listed on the appropriate page. In this way, all the data on projects is always in the same place for easy access.

Carefully analyze your own network goals by drawing your current network and drawing a network you will need in the immediate future. This implies that you have carefully thought out a career path and know where you want to be, say five years from now. Unfortunately, research suggests that women are less able to identify where their career path will lead in five years than men. Women often "back into" their career and talk about their "luck" in obtaining a job by happening to be in the "right place at the right time by accident." Men more often have carefully identified where they want to go professionally and how they will get there. By charting the network you will need you will force yourself to identify more specifically where you want to be in your professional discipline and begin to know how to go about getting there. Design a time table for yourself that identifies what contacts you need to make by what date in order to accomplish a specific career objective. One of the best ways to develop a time table is to work backwards. In other words, start by identifying where and when you want to end up and work backward to the present time. For example, let's say you want your immediate supervisor's job (or one like it in another department) within the next three years. This implies that you have carefully analyzed your career path and have talked with knowledgeable others to determine your qualifications and needed skills to advance. From this analysis you have determined that there are two major areas you need to develop: supervisory skills and budget management. Who are the individuals in your organization who could begin to give you assistance with learning about budget management? What can you do for your boss so she in turn will be willing to turn over some responsibility for budgets? Who can you talk to to find out what projects in the organization need leadership? Can you then volunteer to manage one no one else seems to want to bother with and thus gain experience supervising the work of others? Make a list of the people who will form your new personal network and work backward from the time at which you hope to have accomplished your career objective.

A companion to analyzing your career path is the development of *marketing strategies* for yourself. How do you go about "selling" your own skills and abilities? What did you talk about at the last meeting you attended? Did you let others know what you are doing? Do you have business cards handy to give to people you meet in any setting? Look for ways to make your name familiar and associated with professional competence. You must develop a marketing campaign as carefully as any company develops an advertising program for a new product. Think of one person whose good opinion of you could conceivably work instant magic on your career. Now imagine you happen to be sitting next to this person on an hour long airplane ride. What will you say about yourself?

Finally, *follow-up* every lead, every contact with any potential. If you tell someone you will help them get information, don't fail them. If you indicate that you know someone they should meet, be sure to put them in contact with each other. You never know when failing to follow up on something that may seem of small consequence now could turn into a valuable contact for you later. The chart on the following page summarizes your steps to networking.

If you look at the chart on the next page you will notice that building a network depends on a few key steps: assessing carefully what you want from participation in a network by determining the objectives of your network (will a formal network that you help establish within your own organization better serve you or will your own personal, private network be most useful?), planning the structure of either your own network or a formal network, and following a few "golden rules." No matter what the specific structure or makeup of your network, the integrating ingredient is the *development of a supportive communication climate* between yourself and your fellow networkers. Initially you will need to work at building your fellow colleague's *trust* in your ability and willingness to help them just as much as you want and need their help. If others perceive you as manipulative they will not share information with you

DEVELOPING A NETWORK

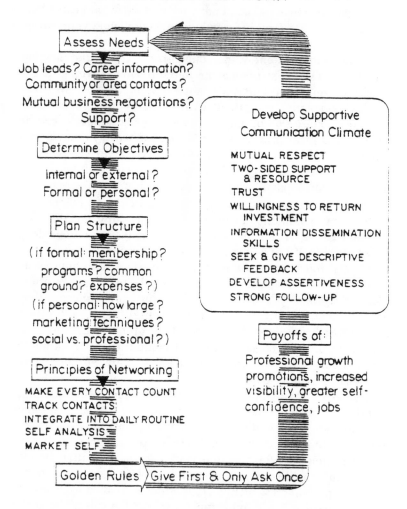

Assess Needs

Job leads? Career information?
Community or area contacts?
Mutual business negotiations?
Support?

Determine Objectives

Internal or external?
Formal or personal?

Plan Structure

(if formal: membership?
programs? common
ground? expenses?)
(if personal: how large?
marketing techniques?
social vs. professional?)

Principles of Networking

MAKE EVERY CONTACT COUNT
TRACK CONTACTS
INTEGRATE INTO DAILY ROUTINE
SELF ANALYSIS
MARKET SELF

Develop Supportive
Communication Climate

MUTUAL RESPECT
TWO-SIDED SUPPORT
  & RESOURCE
TRUST
WILLINGNESS TO RETURN
  INVESTMENT
INFORMATION DISSEMINATION
  SKILLS
SEEK & GIVE DESCRIPTIVE
  FEEDBACK
DEVELOP ASSERTIVENESS
STRONG FOLLOW-UP

Payoffs of:

Professional growth
promotions, increased
visibility, greater self-
confidence, jobs

Golden Rules) Give First & Only Ask Once

for fear that you may one day use it against them. You must be
willing to "return your investment" to the network by *helping
others professionally in the same ways that your career has
been helped.* You will need to develop your *ability to disseminate information* effectively and accurately. Nothing is more
frustrating than for someone to tell you that they have good information for you that turns out to be worthless because you

got it too late or inaccurately. Using *"descriptive feed-back"* means being able to interact with fellow networkers without evaluating or psychologically analyzing their behavior but providing a sounding board for their ideas. By describing their behavior rather than judging it as right or wrong, good or bad, you are much more likely to develop strong reciprocal links. To be successful as a networker and in marketing yourself you will need to *be assertive*. If you are interested in professional growth and in networking, you cannot afford to be shy about asking for help, support, information, or leads. Nor can you hesitate to offer that type of support to others. You will need enough self confidence so that when others reject your offer of help or your request for help, you are not discouraged but simply move on to other contacts.

There are risks in networking. The risk of rejection by others and the unknown quantity that comes from career promotions. I personally feel the risks are worth the potential payoffs of: increased professional growth, promotions, more challenging jobs, increased visibility and greater self-confidence. In order to be successful a networker must be alert to potential contacts, for as one networker put it, "You must fertilize the entire crop because you never know which seeds will germinate." If you are ready to accept the risks of networking in order to generate new challenges in your career, then begin by identifying which "seeds" may germinate from the interactions you have planned for the next 24 hours. Networking begins immediately.